How Are You Fat *and* Saved?

BY SIDDIQU MUHAMMAD

How Are You Fat *and* Saved?

© 2012 by Siddiqu Muhammad

All Rights Reserved

All rights reserved. No part of this publication may be reproduced, stored in a retrieval system or transmitted in any way by any means, electronic, mechanical, photocopy, recording or otherwise, without the prior permission of the author, except as provided by USA copyright law.

ISBN: 978-1-60414-534-2

Acknowledgements and Thank Yous

First off, I have to thank God, who is the head of my life. Without him, nothing would be possible.

Others who deserve my thanks are:

Kyahna Haine who was really supportive in the writing of this book and my inspiration for many of the chapters.

My big brother in the faith, Malachi Israel, who is always sharpening my double-edged sword.

All my brothers Gene aka Big Sexy (Pause), Cordell, Cliff aka Young Gunna, Clerence, Tony aka TJ, Chedane, Kenny, Kwaku. Donnie aka Pro-Blak you always stay holding me down.

There is an entire group that assisted with the book: Jenny Baker, Neela Malover, Dora Dozier, Crystal Tucker (R.I.P Mr. Tucker) Antonia "B-real" Johnson, and Carmen and Lamar Murphy want to send a big huge skinny thank you to you all.

Special thanks to Janelle Hughes for proofreading most of the chapters.

My two favorite sisters, Ayanna and Halimah Muhammad (only two sisters).

My nieces and nephews, Jahad, Jahmal, Dyana, Danay.

My big brother, Asad Muhammad.

My mother, who probably won't read this book either, her husband, Abdual (good brother).

Diana Muhammad, you didn't make the last one but had to shout you out, go change the dance world for the better.

Everything I write is for Zahrah and my father, Siddiqu Muhammad. I took his name so it can live on and stay on everybody's lips.

Also to Valencia and Laci Ward, my aunts and uncle, my Grandmother and Grandfather!

I'm at too many churches to name just one: Full Gospel Christian Assembly International (Church Home), New Joy Divine, Truth and Deliverance, and Victory Christian International.

Author's Note

I wrote an article in 2008 called *"Do Fat People Go to Heaven"* and in the article I cited a study that was done out of Purdue University regarding obesity in the church. The study found that church-goers in general weighed more than the general population. With obesity being the biggest health problem facing us in the 21st Century, I found that to be a very interesting find, for the most part I knew it, but still found it interesting. I eluded in the article to the point that the Bible speaks animatedly against gluttony and eating too much food, yet it's a common practice amongst the Christian community.

I wrote a follow up article in 2010 called *"Would Jesus Jog"* where I touched on the dietary choices of the disciples and how the Bible speaks on physical food and spiritual food being connected. Anyone who attends church on the regular, especially church in the black community, already knew that the body of Christ was an extremely out of shape body. Any given Sunday just walk into a service, and you will first see an overweight usher directing you to your seat, next you will see an overweight musician playing music, then an overweight choir director with an amazing voice singing, only to be followed up by an out of shape preacher giving the word of God.

For a personal trainer you almost want to ask, "Are we promoting God or fast food?" The "why" is very much common knowledge as well. After church service you can find an array of cakes, pies, snacks, and fried chicken dinners, not to mention church is one of the only places where the bigger you are the more you are loved. Culturally we can see this in every single Tyler Perry or Christian based movie. The most overweight character is the character that is usually the most sought after for knowledge, wisdom, and understanding.

The Bible is not only very clear on obesity being one of the worst sins one can perform against God and themselves, but the Bible also provides the solution to the problem. Sitting under Apostle Aaron Royster, Apostle Ron Wilson, Apostle John T. Abercrombie, Pastor Curtis Hill who are all highly regarded men of God, has given me the insight and fortitude to write this extremely controversial but long overdue book.

How are you Fat* and *Saved? is the blueprint for physical wellbeing in the body of Christ and as my spiritual big brother and cousin Malachi Israel would say, *"A must-read for anyone who calls themselves a Christian."*

God healing the sick is a highly regarded miracle in scripture. It is called *Divine Healing* within the church. *Divine Health* is also a miracle in the scripture but is often overlooked. *Divine Health* is where a believer is so aligned with the will of God that they don't fall victim to sickness and disease. The latter is much more appealing but the "how" has to be taught.

"How, then, can they call on the one they have not believed in? And how can they believe in the one of whom they have not heard? And how can they hear without someone preaching to

them? And how can they preach unless they are sent? As it is written, "How beautiful are the feet of those who bring good news!"

ROMANS 10:14-15

Take a walk with me through the scriptures of God and allow his spirit to direct your future choices as I allowed his spirit to direct mine. This book was extremely difficult for me to write because I knew it would offend many people, but I would rather offend people and save their life than not to. God is very forgiving and very merciful and like any parent, wants only the best for his offspring. Hear what God has to say about exercise and eating from the mouths of his prophets and messengers. As believers let's be torchlight's for the world. The first way to be that is by representing a physical manifestation of what God would have a believer do. **Be Fit 4 Christ.**

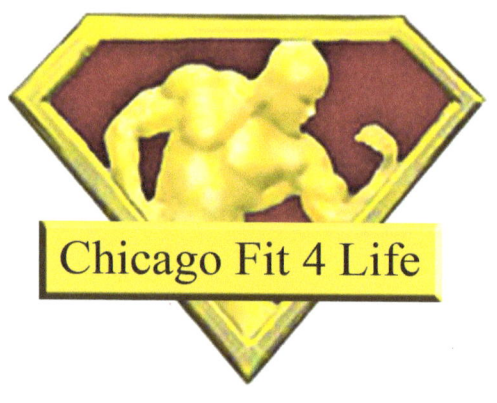

Table of Contents

Acknowledgements and Thank Yous 3
Author's Note v

The Problem 1
   KINGDOM BUILDING 2
   WHO IS YOUR GOD? 3

Fasting 7
   WHAT IS FASTING? 8
   SUPERNATURAL WEIGHT LOSS 11
   TYPES OF FASTS 13

PERSONAL STORY #1 — Nikita Randle 20

The Garden 23
   THE ELEMENTS OF LIFE 24
   BENEFITS FROM FRUITS AND VEGETABLES 24

PERSONAL STORY #2 — Kyahna Haine 32

Forbidden Fruit 35
   SATAN'S FIRST LIE 36
   CLEAN VS UNCLEAN 38
   OLD TESTAMENT VS. NEW TESTAMENT: 40
   THE SINS OF THE FATHER 44

Would a man rob God? 51
   PRICE/COST/WORTH 54

PERSONAL STORY #3 — Talyia 58

Building Solomon's Temple 61
    TYPES OF EXERCISE 63

BONUS CHAPTERS

Water —the liquid of life 78
Sleep is the Cousin of Death 86
Under the Influence 89

How Are You Fat *and* Saved?

The Problem

"Be not among drunkards or among gluttonous eaters of meat, for the drunkard and the glutton will come to poverty, and slumber will clothe them with rags."

PROVERBS 23:20-21

The Church is the fattest and most out of shape institution on earth! Week after week in churches around the United States, you'll find sermons being preached on morality, prosperity, and a list of other issues facing the community. One issue that isn't discussed is health and weight of the congregants. Yet this issue is the most important issue in the spreading of the Gospel. How can I make a bold declaration like this?

{A study by Northwestern University researchers concludes that young adults who are regularly involved in religious activities have a significantly higher chance of becoming obese by middle age. And the results are of special concern to black women, who are some of the most dedicated churchgoers.}

{A study published by Purdue University Professor Ken Ferraro examined the relationships between religion and both

body mass index (BMI) and obesity. *The study found that church members tend to be more overweight than the general population, and Baptists, including Southern Baptists, have the distinction of being the most overweight religious group in the study.}*

KINGDOM BUILDING

Well for one, if members aren't healthy then they cannot contribute anything to the development of Kingdom Building. Have you noticed how health has a way of putting things into perspective, while at the same time limiting what one can do?

Take the billionaire business tycoon for instance. He owns cars, jets, and houses all over the world, yet when he receives news that he has been stricken with cancer all he can think about is preserving his own life. The only thing that matters to him is his health. He isn't at fault for immediately changing his priorities; self-preservation is the first law of nature. The church is more to blame for not informing people on what will take place if you mistreat God's most precious house, the human body.

A pastor wants to increase the membership of his church, but the pastor and the members are overweight. Before anyone can hear words coming from one's mouth, they see the person who is giving the word. When seeing a person, a list of assumptions is formulated in one's mind (lazy, dumb, out of shape, easily tempted, etc...)

Before speaking on how much you love God, a person of sound mind will always think, **"how can you love God and you don't even love yourself?"** The human body is a temporary gift that is given by God. How one treats one's self is directly related to their faith in God.

WHO IS YOUR GOD?

"Do you not know that your body is a temple of the Holy Spirit, who is in you, whom you have received from God? You are not your own!"

1 CORINTHIANS 6:19

Even though being in shape and being fit makes a person physically look better, that is only a very small focus of exercise and healthy eating. Looking better is the results of adopting a healthy lifestyle but there are so many other reasons to adopt one.

The obesity epidemic is at an all-time high worldwide. According to the Center for Disease Control over 50% of the US population is overweight and/or obese. That number amongst Christians is drastically higher.

Walk into a church in Atlanta, Chicago, Montgomery, or any city or small town on a Sunday and tell me what you see, then not only look at what you see listen to what is being prayed. *"Let's say an extra prayer for Ms. Johnson she is in the hospital for heart failure, again"* How about we take up a collection to hire Ms. Johnson a personal trainer and a nutritionist! Ms. Johnson is eating herself to death and if we want to save her life let's look in her kitchen.

Look at what's being served after service (fried chicken, peach cobbler, candy). I actually speak at Churches that have candy shops right in the lobby. With the majority of their congregation being diabetic, that can't be a good idea. That's like having a bar in the lobby of the Church and the majority of your congregation is alcoholic.

How can the Church expect God to bless us when we have obviously forgone his first commandment? Exodus 20:3 "You shall have no other gods before Me."

"Wait a second Siddiqu, I thought we were talking about poor health, not exercising, and being fat?"

If you eat 5 times a day, yet you pray 2 times a day, then I know what "God" you serve and put your faith in. It is not the creator of the heavens and earth. It's more like the creator of the Big Mac and fries. (Sorry I didn't see your foot right there) John 10:10 *"... I came that they may have life and have it abundantly."*

The word Abundance means extremely plentiful or over sufficient quantity. By definition, one cannot have an abundance of life without an abundance of health. Here's a short list of some of the ailments that are the by-product of being overweight:

- High blood cholesterol, dyslipidemia
- Insulin resistance, glucose intolerance
- Congestive heart failure
- Gout
- Osteoarthritis
- Some types of cancer (such as endometrial, breast, prostate, and colon)
- Complications of pregnancy
- Poor female reproductive health (such as menstrual irregularities, infertility, irregular ovulation)
- Bladder control problems (such as stress incontinence)
- Psychological disorders (such as depression, eating disorders, distorted body image, and low self-esteem)

Obesity is the fastest growing health risk in America. **In 2003, the Center For Disease Control declared obesity as the most serious health risk facing this country.** As Christians, we are supposed to be an example for the world, a beacon of light for hope in a world of despair. So, when the world is facing a crisis it comes to the church for the solution.

What is the Body of Christ doing for its very own body? Not much! The church is part of the problem and the problem has been swept underneath a rug for far too long. There is an elephant in the room and that elephant is called Christians!

> *"But I say, walk by the Spirit,
> and you will not carry out the desire of the flesh."*
>
> GAL. 5:16

Christians are unhealthy because they are living in a carnal mind and therefore producing a body that is not atheistically pleasing and filled with poor health. I have searched the Bible from Genesis to Revelation and found that God did not leave the believer with an empty hand and an oversized stomach. He knew this problem would come and he gave us multiple solutions to face it.

Poor health and growing waistlines isn't the end all be all, it's just a way for God to manifest his greatness and glory. God made our bodies so he had to give us an instructional manual on how to maintain them and what to do in a case of emergency. When a person is taking 6 different pills in the morning to stay alive, I would say that is an emergency. When a person has a difficult time sitting down and standing up, I would say that is an emergency. It is now time for Christians to go to their emergency manual and follow the instructions. The real problem is that believers are not taking heed to the instructions and allowing the world to dictate how they live. We are allowing the world to come up with solutions to a problem that they created, (i.e. Jenny Craig, Atkins Diet, weight loss pills, etc…)

The time has come for believers to say, *"Enough is enough, I will not live to eat but rather eat to live. If God so loved the world that he gave his only begotten son, then I should not have any attachments to foods or any schedule that won't allow my very own life to be my priority."*

> *"If you are a big eater, put a knife to your throat;"*
>
> PROVERBS 23:2

Fasting

"You have to be more hungry for the things of the spirit than you are a piece a meat"

—DR. CREFLO DOLLAR

"Yet when they were ill, I put on sackcloth and humbled myself with fasting. When my prayers returned to me unanswered,"

—PSALM 35:13

Fasting is and always has been the secret weapon of the believer. To want to lose weight and not give up any amount of food is a ridiculous concept, the equivalent to ***spiritual welfare.*** God doesn't give out link cards; you link up with God and watch your desire for the flesh dissipates. The idea of something for nothing is anti-God and easily exploited by Satan.

Billions of dollars go into the weight loss industry every year with Christians rushing to products that promise them a gorgeous body with no work. *"Lose 30 pounds in 30 days and eat as many cookies as you want!"*

In the book of Leviticus, Chapter 16: Verse 29, it explains that fasting is the same as "afflicting one's soul." *Yep, you read that last sentence correctly.* If there is a struggle in your financial life, put yourself on a fast. If your marriage is in shambles and on the rocks, put yourself on a fast and ask your spouse to do the same. ***If you are overweight and out of shape — get on a fast and do it fast!***

My life's work is to make sure every believer is walking in divine health and only tapping into divine healing as a last resort. Since it's very clear that most believers are not walking anywhere, I'm equally clear on the reason why — they are eating themselves to death by eating too much food and too much of the wrong foods.

THINK ABOUT IT

An obese Christian woman once told me she didn't eat too much food and always ate the right food; she just ate at the wrong time.

I told her, "I didn't know *always* was a time!"

We serve such a merciful God that he actually gave us a weapon to fight against the problem of obesity; Fasting.

WHAT IS FASTING?

The Greek derivative of the word "fast" is **nestia**. It means, "not to eat food." Fasting can also be looked at as the restraint from something to redirect your focus on where it should be, God. Eating food is a very natural act; it's so natural that every single human being in existence does it. Babies eat, teenagers eat, a person in the hospital will still manage to eat food even if it's very little.

Denying yourself food amplifies what you are trying to do in the presence of God. Christians have to move past the days of just saying, *"I want to lose weight... I want to be healthier... I want to play with my grandchildren and even live long enough to see my daughter married off..."* We have to show God we really desire what we profess from our lips.

As a trainer I meet so many people of faith who claim they really want to lose weight, but they just don't know how. When I suggest that they should stop eating, I always get the same confused look. A look that says, *"Have you lost your mind? If I stop eating I will die."*

News flash Christian Community: You have already died and are now *born again* as a new creature in Christ. Secondly, you still must die a physical death in this world. Thirdly, you are killing yourself faster by eating than you ever will if you stop eating.

If you drop the "T" in diet, that is what the majority of Christians are doing when they pull up to the drive thru, stash that bag of cookies in there drawer at work or create a secret candy stash in their bedroom.

THINK ABOUT IT

The first person to fast in the Bible was Moses. He set the bar for every believer and showed what can be done with the denial of one's self for the greater whole.

> *"And he was there with the LORD forty days and forty nights; he did neither eat bread, nor drink water. And he wrote upon the tables the words of the covenant, the Ten Commandments."*
>
> — EXODUS 34:28

Through Moses giving up bread and wine for 40 days and 40 nights, he was able to create the Ten Commandments. Ask yourself what you can create if you did the same? There is a desire in anyone who is overweight to lose weight, or anyone who takes medicine to get off of medicine.

No matter how much the media tries to push the big/beautiful campaigns an overweight/obese person is never truly comfortable when they are at their heaviest. There must be sense of fairness as we approach this; if a person doesn't want to give up anything do they really deserve God's assistance?

Would you really ask God to heal/change you, but you plan on eating all the same greasy foods, all the same snacks, and not exercise at all? The mere arrogance of this type of backwards thinking is enough to completely see why the Christian community leads in every major obesity related preventable disease.

THINK ABOUT IT

Fasting is a sacrifice. Sacrifice means giving up something you love for something that you love more.

My mother taught me as a child, *"Anything worth having is worth fighting for"* One must ask the question, *"Is your health and longevity worth having?"* If the answer is yes, then it's worth fighting for. The weapon that you will use is a weapon that has been used by everyone who has embarked on a lifestyle change, and that is FASTING!

> *"And I set my face unto the Lord God, to seek by prayer and supplications, with fasting, and sackcloth, and ashes: And I prayed unto the Lord God, and made my confession..."*
>
> — DANIEL 9:34

SUPERNATURAL WEIGHT LOSS

God gave Christians fasting as a means of creating miracles in their life. Food is natural; you realize that it is natural because you don't have to be taught to desire food. By giving up something natural, you immediately place yourself in the realm of a supernatural being. A supernatural believer can create supernatural results in their life.

When a client asks me, *"How much weight should I lose a week?"*

I tell them, *"One to two pounds a week is the ideal rate of weight loss."*

If the person isn't really serious, he or she will say "that's too slow" and attempt some shortcut to weight loss — surgery, pills, starvation, etc.... They never really take the time to do the math and realize what those numbers truly represent.

- One pound a week adds up to over 50 pounds in a year.
- Two pounds a week adds up to more than 100 pounds in a year.

Weight loss like this means a person can go from being obese to being underweight in one year's time. A 5'5" woman who weighs 225 pounds and has a body fat percentage of 35% is obese. A 5'5 woman who is 125 pounds with a body fat percentage of 14% is really thin and in many circles considered too skinny.

That weight loss outlined above could mean that the above description is of the same woman! That is a <u>miracle</u>! For a woman to go from being considered obese to being considered too skinny in one year's time is amazing.

Notice I did not say in one *day's* time. This woman didn't take one day to put the weight on, so it won't take her one day to get it off.

The discipline that a person would need to accomplish losing 100 pounds in a year is readily available with fasting.

The word "miracle" derives from the word "mira" which means to wonder at.

When you know someone who was out of shape/overweight and you see him or her and they've lost the weight, what is the first question you ask? *"How did you do it?"* How they did it is something that you wondered at.

The process is simple, but because it has become so uncommon, you have to ask questions like, *"Did you hire a trainer? What did you take out of your diet? What kept you motivated? ..."*

You wonder how they changed the way they look. You understand they had to change something, because it's not natural to *look* different without *doing* something different.

> **"Then they all came and urged David to eat something while it was still day; but David took an oath, saying, "May God deal with me, be it ever so severely, if I taste bread or anything else before the sun sets!"**
>
> —2 SAMUEL 3:35

The biggest FEAR (False Evidence Appearing Real) with fasting is that a person will be too hungry to continue with his or her daily tasks. When was the last time you experienced a hunger for God so strong that you were unable to function at work? Where you thirsted and hungered for his "word," where you couldn't wait until Sunday and had to stop everything and shut out everybody so you could get closer to him? Most people will say, "I have never been to the point where I can't function because of my hunger for God and his word, and the reason is because God created us to have a balanced life."

This means he wouldn't allow us to fast if he felt we would be unable to function while doing it. Fasting is not a commandant in the New Testament. The reason for that is God wants Christians to *want* to deny themselves. He doesn't want to force an individual who is born again to make sacrifices for Him.

John 3:16: *"God so loved the world that he gave his only begotten son..."*

He did that for you, can't you at least give up a little food for a short period of time? It sounds easy in theory, but I have a question for all the "True Believers" out there. *Do you fast on a regular basis?* Better yet, *What is a regular basis?*

For argument's sake, let's say a regular basis is once a month. *Do you fast once a month? Any type of fast?*

**"And he said unto them,
This kind can come forth by nothing, but by prayer and fasting."**

— MARK 9:29

TYPES OF FASTS

When I discuss fasting here, I want you to understand we are talking about taking something out of your life for a limited period of time. At least once a week, usually Sunday, I go without food or drink until about 6pm. Why do I do this? Well for one reason, I attend Church service on Sunday at **Full Gospel Christian Assembly International**. When I sit under my spiritual leader, I believe that the words that will come forth from his mouth will be life-changing every time.

When going under certain surgeries the doctor will ask the patient to go without food or drink for 24 hours. *Why?* Because the procedures that will be taking place are life-changing and food in one's systems can disrupt the surgery.

In the same say, any spiritual leader's voice that I am under on Sunday is God performing surgery on my spirit, soul, and body and I don't want food to disrupt the operation.

There are many different types of fasts. Here is a short list of a few.

> *"In those days I, Daniel, was mourning three full weeks. I ate no pleasant food, no meat or wine came into my mouth, nor did I anoint myself at all, till three whole weeks were fulfilled."*
>
> — DANIEL 10:2,3

DANIEL FAST — FRUIT & VEGETABLE FAST

This is a fast where foods that are grown from the earth is ones complete diet. The reason this fast is such a good fast to be on, is because this is the closest to the diet that Adam and Eve were on before there fall.

The Daniel fast is a diet that God wants all human beings to strive for. It has been shown in science to produce a body for longevity and an abundance of life. There is no proof that a human should die at 75, 100, or even 125 years of age. It is not known how long a person can stay alive, but removing meat and wine from ones diet, even for a short period of time can do nothing but assist in longevity.

While on the Daniel Fast, try to eat only organic fruits and vegetables.

THINK ABOUT IT

The average conventionally-grown apple has 20-30 artificial poisons on its skin, even after rinsing. Organic produce also contains on average 50% more vitamins, minerals, enzymes and other micro-nutrients than intensively farmed produce.

Foods to include in your diet during the Daniel Fast

FRUITS — these can be fresh, frozen, dried, juiced or canned. Fruits include but are not limited to apples, apricots, bananas, blackberries, blueberries, cantaloupe, cherries, cranberries, dates, figs, grapefruit, grapes, guava, honeydew melon, kiwi, lemons, limes, mangoes, nectarines, oranges, papayas, peaches, pears, pineapples, plums, prunes, raisins, raspberries, strawberries, tangelos, tangerines, watermelon

VEGETABLES — these can be fresh, frozen, dried, juiced or canned. Vegetables include but are not limited to artichokes, asparagus, beets, broccoli, Brussels sprouts, cabbage, carrots, cauliflower, celery, chili peppers, collard greens, corn, cucumbers, eggplant, garlic, ginger root, kale, leeks, lettuce, mushrooms, mustard greens, okra, onions, parsley, potatoes, radishes, rutabagas, scallions, spinach, sprouts, squashes, sweet potatoes, tomatoes, turnips, watercress, yams, zucchini, veggie burgers are an option if you are not allergic to soy.

WHOLE GRAINS — including but not limited to whole wheat, brown rice, millet, quinoa, oats, barley, grits, whole wheat pasta, whole wheat tortillas, rice cakes and popcorn.

NUTS AND SEEDS — including but not limited to sunflower seeds, cashews, peanuts, sesame. Also nut butters including peanut butter.

LEGUMES — these can be canned or dried. Legumes include but are not limited to dried beans, pinto beans, split peas, lentils, kidney beans, black beans, cannelloni beans, Navy beans.

OILS — including but not limited to olive, canola, grape seed, peanut, and sesame.

BEVERAGES — only be spring water, distilled water or other pure waters.

Foods to Avoid on the Daniel Fast

MEAT AND ANIMAL PRODUCTS — including but not limited to beef, lamb, pork, poultry, and fish.

DAIRY — including but not limited to milk, cheese, cream, butter, and eggs.

SWEETENERS — including but not limited to sugar, raw sugar, honey, syrups, molasses, and cane juice.

ALL BREADS — including but not limited to barely, wheat, rye, white.

REFINED AND PROCESSED FOOD PRODUCTS — including but not limited to artificial flavorings, food additives, chemicals, white foods — white rice, white flour, and foods that contain artificial preservatives.

DEEP FRIED FOODS — including but not limited to potato chips, French fries, corn chips.

SOLID FATS — including shortening, margarine, lard and foods high in fat.

BEVERAGES — including but not limited to coffee, tea, herbal teas, carbonated beverages, energy drinks, and alcohol.

> *"On the tenth day of the appointed month in early autumn, you must deny yourselves. Neither native-born Israelites nor foreigners living among you may do any kind of work. This is a permanent law for you."*
>
> — LEVITICUS 16:29

LEVITICUS FAST OR ABSOLUTE FAST

This is a fast where you deny yourself everything including water. This fast is one that has to be limited on time. I would not suggest a person go over two days with an absolute fast. You also cannot do an absolute fast unless you have showed an extreme level of discipline with any of the other fast, because it is the most difficult. This is also a fast that could be better performed during an off day from work if one has a physically taxing job. Make sure you are reading your Bible during this fast; the word of God will offset your hunger pains.

WATER FAST

This is a fast where you only drink water and eat NO food. I've read that 75% of American are dehydrated and do not know it. If this number is correct then this fast breeds so many benefits. Water is mentioned in the Bible 722 times. I will go into the importance of water later on in this book, but for now just understand that it is essential to life.

Perform this fast from Sun up to sunset, and eat a dinner that is not greasy and stacked with vegetables. There are so many distractions that come into a person's life on a daily basis that by drinking just water one's mind becomes sharper and more attuned to God's voice.

Did believers fast?

- Moses fasted for forty days and forty nights, twice back-to-back, without food or water, the first, immediately before he received the tablets on the mountain with God. And the second, after coming down, seeing the Israelites practicing idolatry, and breaking the tablets in anger.
- King David fasted when the son of his adulterous union with Bathsheba was struck sick by God in punishment for the adultery and for David's murder of Bathsheba's husband, Uriah the Hittite. David used fasting as an act of humbling his soul.
- King Jehoshaphat proclaimed a fast throughout Judah for victory over the Moabites and Ammonites who were attacking them.
- Prophet Joel called for a fast to avert the judgment of God. The people of Nineveh, in response to Jonah's prophecy, fasted to avert the judgment of God.
- [a] Queen Esther declared a three-day fast for all the Jews prior to risking her life in visiting King Ahasuerus uninvited.

- The prophetess Anna, who proclaimed the baby Jesus to be the Messiah, prayed and fasted regularly in the Temple.
- Jesus fasted for forty days and forty nights while in the desert, being tempted by Satan to turn stones into bread and eat them, among other temptations. Jesus teaches on the outward appearance and demeanor of a fasting person.
- Paul did not eat or drink anything for three days after he converted on the road to Damascus. The church in Antioch were worshipping the Lord and fasting when the Holy Spirit told them to send Barnabas and Paul for work. Paul and Barnabus went on to appoint elders with prayer and fasting.

PERSONAL STORY #1

Nikita Randle

CHURCH: New Faith Baptist Church International
PASTOR: Rev. Dr. Trunell D. Felder

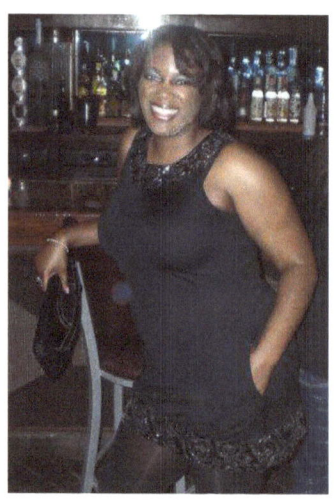

BEFORE

Nikita Randle was a young woman with an athletic background. She ran track and played on the volleyball team in high school, which kept Kita slim and trim through college. After graduating from college, things changed for her — and the change was drastic!

Kita took a job that required her to travel a lot. This meant eating at restaurants for every meal, every day. The job gave her an American Express card for "traveling expenses" and she made sure she got her money's worth.

Have you ever ordered more food than normal or chosen "fancy" fatty foods you wouldn't normally eat at a restaurant just because someone else was picking up the tab? Well, that's what Kita did Monday through Friday for a year straight! She was thriving professionally and it showed in her waistline, at the end of her yearlong extravaganza, she had gained 30 pounds!

Those 30 pounds caused her to go up three dress sizes. Buying new clothes to all of the time to accommodate her ever-expanding size was costly, too.

One of Kita's close friends had recently become engaged, and Kita didn't feel good about going to the wedding being. She knew she was now cute in the face but wide in the waist. She'd tried diet plans in the past but most did nothing but take a few pounds off, only to have them come right back again.

She grew tired of fluctuating in weight and made her goal to get down to "bikini size" and stay there until she had children. Kita contacted me, her good friend Siddiqu Muhammad, to assist her with this challenge. When she contacted me, she sent a one-sentence text message that simply read, "I want my sexy back!"

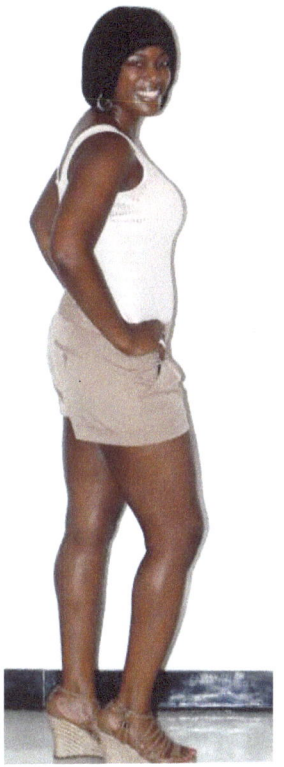

AFTER

I knew exactly what the text meant and what needed to be done. Kita was instantly put on strict diet plant that consisted mostly of fruits and vegetables. She dedicated herself to exercising almost every day of the week. We're not talking about a 30 minute stroll or a leisurely ride on the bike, either. She was in the toughest aerobic and cycling classes and I pushed her to the limit as often as I could.

Sometimes I would make her perform exercises until I got tired of watching, while constantly reminding her about "getting her sexy back!" Kita was losing two to three pounds a week, and she reached her goal within 4 months. The way she did this was by making up her mind and going for it! It's like Kita always says, ***"The scale doesn't weigh your excuses."***

KITA'S WEEKLY EXERCISE ROUTINE:

MONDAY: Boot Camp
TUESDAY: Cycling
WEDNESDAY: Body works plus abs
THURSDAY: Personal Training session
FRIDAY: Rest
SATURDAY: Cycling
SUNDAY: Personal Training session

KITA'S DIET OPTIONS:

BREAKFAST:
- oatmeal with raisins and brown sugar
- red apple and plum
- red apple and banana

LUNCH:
- salmon
- tuna salad

SNACK:
- Strawberry Special K

DINNER:
- fresh cut vegetables (yellow squash, zucchini, onion, and mushrooms/seasoned with Mrs. Dash)
- tuna salad
- Tilapia with fresh spinach (cooked)

The Garden

Then God said, "I give you every seed-bearing plant on the face of the whole earth and every tree that has fruit with seed in it. They will be yours for food."

— GENESIS 1:29

As I've toured churches speaking on exercise and fitness, I've found that one question always comes up: *"Are fruits and vegetables good for you? ... Because I heard...* fruits have too much sugar and cause blood sugar problems, eating too much fruit will give you an overdose of potassium, eating fruit causes cancer, etc.

The Christian community cannot afford to buy into rhetoric regarding fruits and vegetables when the scripture clearly informs believers about how important they are to one's diet. Adam and Eve were created in a garden and given eternal life. They eventually lost their position and would experience a physical death not because of a dietary choice but because of disobedience to God's will. While in the garden they had a specific diet, a diet that consisted of foods that can only be grown, not manufactured and not killed.

The elements of life

A garden produces fruit, which is the edible part of a plant, and vegetables, which are plants, that are edible. There are so many other foods believers should take out of their diets before removing fruits and vegetables. These are some of the only foods that will never come in packages or containers, and they are foods that God himself made.

Many believers understand how healthy these foods are for them, but they don't know now much of their diets should be made up of fruits and vegetables. A diet high in fruits and vegetables reduces one's risk of cancer, Type 2 Diabetes, hypertension, and a long list of other health problems. They also help stave off things such as obesity, stomach ulcers, acne, and on and on!

Fruits and vegetables not only help to prolong your life, but help improve the overall quality of life. You've heard the saying, *"An apple a day keeps the doctor away."* Most of you don't take that saying literally enough. The reality of the situation is an apple does help you stay out of the doctor's office for anything from sleep apnea to the common cold. Fruits and vegetables affect the human body in such a healing way because they are high in vitamins, minerals and fiber — and they're low in calories.

BENEFITS FROM FRUITS AND VEGETABLES
- **Vitamins** — The word vitamin is made up of two parts — "vita" meaning life and "amine" meaning contains nitrogen. The human body requires vitamins in order to function. Different vitamins perform different jobs, but they all work together for the common good. For example, *Vitamin A* promotes eyesight and helps us see in the dark, and *Vitamin K* helps blood clot, etc. Collectively there are 13 different vita-

mins. Some are fat-soluble, which means your body uses fat to absorb them; and some water-soluble, which means your body uses water to absorb them.

- **Minerals** — These are pure inorganic elements containing atoms of the same element, meaning they are much simpler in chemical form than vitamins. All vitamins are required in order for the body to function properly, but not all minerals are required. Some minerals are necessary at one stage of life, but not at another. For example, the mineral *calcium* aids in osteoporosis prevention and *iron* in preventing iron-deficiency or anemia.

- **Fiber** — This virtually indigestible substance helps keep your weight under control by making you feel full and by helping to move old, decaying food from your system. Fiber can absorb large amounts of water in the bowels, and this makes stools softer and easier to pass. About three different times a year, my clients and I go on a three-day all-fruit and vegetable fast. Each time someone performs the fast for the first time, they comment on how light they feel afterward because they have eliminated all of that old waste.

Eating fewer calories has been proven to lead to an abundance (more than enough) of life. A calorie-restricted diet provides all the nutrients necessary for a healthy life, but minimizes the energy (calories) supplied in the diet. This type of diet increases the life span of mice and delays the onset of age-related chronic diseases such as cancers, heart disease, and stroke in rodents.

— FROM A STUDY BY ANTHONY CIVITARESE, ERIC RAVUSSIN, AND COLLEAGUES (PENNINGTON BIOMEDICAL RESEARCH CENTER).

ADDING FRUITS AND VEGETABLES TO YOUR DIET

Fruits and vegetables won't just jump onto your plate and into your mount. You need to incorporate them in your diet, and that takes some work.

> *And the LORD God commanded the man,*
> *"You are free to eat from any tree in the garden"*
>
> — GENESIS 2:16

Making a lifestyle change means actually *changing* something in your life. Here are a few suggestions for how to start incorporating more fruits and vegetables into your diet:

- **BUY FRUIT** — This may seem pretty obvious, but many of us never take the time to plan what we're going to shop for before we go to the store. I had a client who couldn't lose any weight because she kept eating the wrong foods that were already in her pantry. She hadn't been grocery shopping for new foods that fit her new lifestyle.

- **MAKE FRUITS AND VEGETABLES ACCESSIBLE** — If you buy some apples and put them in the fruit storage bin in your refrigerator, an apple probably won't be your first choice as a snack because it's not out where you can see it. I've watched this happen in my own home, and then find spoiled fruit in places I normally never look. Put those fruits and vegetables in the middle of the kitchen table if you have to!

- **MAKE YOUR SNACKS** — Prepare your own snacks and take them to work with you. Making fruits and/or vegetables your go-to snacks means having them available when and where you want to eat snacks. A big motivation for taking the time to do this is that fruits and vegetables have fewer calories and make you feel more full than packaged snacks. For example, one snack-sized bag of corn chips (1 ounce) has the same number of calories as a small apple, one cup of whole strawberries or 1 cup of carrots with 1/4 cup of low-calorie dip. Making substitutions like these each time you snack will leave you feeling more satisfied while you consume fewer calories. Another added bonus is that you might just save money, too.

What do fruits and vegetables do?

Below you will find a list of some fruits and vegetables and what specific affect they have on your health. There seems to be a link between a physical ailment and something in nature to offset it. When Adam and Eve disobeyed the instructions God gave them, they were removed from the garden. The reason they couldn't remain in the Garden was because the Garden represented eternal life and the diet that they would've had inside the garden. While outside the Garden, they had to eat foods that were the opposite of life — foods that represented death.

> *"The tongue has the power of life and death, and those who love it will eat its fruit."*
>
> — PROVERBS 18:21

WILD MIXED BERRIES — Blueberries, raspberries, strawberries, blackberries, cranberries, goji berries, coffee, noni, acai, etc. These berries, as a whole, are nutritional powerhouses filled with antioxidants and nutrients. They can help with joint health, heart health, aid in cancer prevention and help prevent muscular degeneration along with providing a host of other benefits.

KIWIS are an often-overlooked fruit. They look weird and are sometimes out of season. Don't let that deter you. Kiwis have twice the Vitamin C of oranges. Kiwis are one of the most nutrient-dense fruits on the planet. They are high in fiber and potassium for a healthy heart. Kiwis have been shown to not only prevent oxidative DNA damage but also help stimulate the repair of the cellular damage that has occurred.

CHERRIES are loaded with antioxidant compounds that are anti-inflammatory, anti-aging, and anti-cancer. They contain wonderful quercetin, an anti-cancer compound. They also contain ellagic acid, a powerful anti-tumor compound that causes cancer cell death (apoptosis) with no damage to healthy cells. Cherries also contain melatonin, which helps regulate sleep patterns.

POMEGRANATE JUICE, in quantities of just a few ounces everyday, has been proven to lower blood pressure, improve cardiovascular health, and help slow aging. Pomegranates are also shown to help prevent LDL cholesterol oxidation, help prevent blood clotting, slow the growth of prostate cancer, and improve erectile dysfunction.

RED DELICIOUS APPLES have the most antioxidants of any apple, mainly due their deep red color. Apples, like cherries, contain quercetin, which is a powerful natural anti-inflammatory that may help prevent Alzheimer's and heart disease. Apples are also high in pectin, a great soluble shown to help lower LDL cholesterol, and boron, which may help prevent osteoporosis and arthritis

EGGPLANT improves the brain's ability to focus. Eggplant has a compound called *Nasunin* that protects brain cells from damage. It also helps to improve cardiovascular health with its high levels of potassium and fiber.

CARROTS help improve eye, skin, and hair. Carrots are great because they can be cut up and used as a healthy snack to nibble throughout the day. One carrot has enough Vitamin A for an entire day. Carrots can help reduce your risk of having heart disease by up to 60%. Another great benefit from eating carrots is that a large intake of carotenoids can decrease different forms of cancer by up to 50%.

BROCCOLI reduces the risk of stomach, lung, and rectal cancer. Broccoli has a strong, positive impact on our body's detoxification system. It possesses high levels of Vitamin C and folate, which aids in the body's ability to fight off colds, flu, and even allergies.

SWEET POTATOES help to lessen the effects of arthritis and reduce the risk of colon cancer and diabetes. Sweet potatoes may even protect cigarette smokers and those who live with them from emphysema by virtue of its Vitamin A, as cigarette smoke creates a deficiency of this vitamin. This deficiency may be one of the causes of emphysema.

TOMATOES are a metabolism booster. *Lycopene,* a compound found in tomatoes, is renowned for its cancer-fighting capabilities. Studies conducted by Harvard researchers have discovered that men who consumed 10 servings of tomatoes a week, or the equivalent of 10 slices of pizza, can cut the risk of developing prostate cancer by a formidable 45 percent. This vegetable can be used in paste, soup, juice or sauce form for whatever, whenever. Tomatoes are also high in potassium, fiber and Vitamins A & K.

KALE is known for its detoxification ability and its cancer fighting qualities. It has high levels of Vitamin C, folate, and fiber. The fiber-related components in kale do a better job of binding together with bile acids in your digestive tract when they've been steamed. When this binding process takes place, it's easier for bile acids to be excreted, and the result is a lowering of your cholesterol levels.

SAMPLE FRUIT & VEGETABLE DIET OPTIONS:

BREAKFAST:

- ½ orange or (1) 8 ounce glass orange juice or pomegranate juice
- 2 slices of tomatoes
- Water

LUNCH:

- Mixed salad with lettuce, tomatoes, cucumbers, green peppers
- Low fat/low calorie salad dressing
- Water

AFTERNOON SNACK:

- Bowl of blueberries
- 1 apple sliced

DINNER:

- Green Beans
- Broccoli, carrot, cauliflower medley steamed

EVENING SNACK:

- 2 servings raw vegetables

For many, a diet that only consists of fruits and vegetables isn't that appealing. I would agree with those people, but sometimes it's helpful. When you really understand the health benefits of what this type of diet does for your body, you will understand. I would encourage everyone to take time off from any food that isn't a fruit or vegetable for several days. This may seem difficult at first, but it's not impossible, **Philippians 4:13 "I can do everything through Christ who strengthens me."**

Fruits and vegetables never come with an ingredient label on their sides. The reason for this is that God makes them himself. Adam did not create the garden he lived in; he was created in a garden that already existed. This must have meant that God created it. His reason for creating the garden was not only to give Adam a job but also so that Adam could benefit from the rich food that would come forth from the garden. If Adam was to benefit from the food of the Garden, then why shouldn't Christians today benefit from it as well?

SAMPLE FRUIT AND VEGETABLE SALADS:

- Cube watermelon and combine with tomato chunks, basil and basic vinaigrette. You can substitute peach for the watermelon or the tomato. (Not both. Okay?)
- Mix wedges of tomatoes and peaches, add slivers of red onion, a few red-pepper flakes and cilantro. Dress with olive oil and lime or lemon juice.
- Cucumber salad: Slice cucumbers thin (if they're fat and old, peel and seed them first), toss with red onions and salt, then let sit for 20 to 60 minutes. Rinse, dry, dress with cider vinegar mixed with Dijon mustard; no oil necessary.
- Shave raw asparagus stalks with a vegetable peeler. Discard the tough first pass of the peeler — i.e., the peel — but do use the tips, whole. Dress with lemon vinaigrette and coarse salt. (Chopped hard-boiled eggs are an optional but good addition.)
- Grate or very thinly slice Jerusalem artichokes, mix with pitted and chopped oil-cured olives, olive oil, lemon juice and a sprinkling of coarsely ground cumin.

PERSONAL STORY #2

Kyahna Haine

CHURCH: Victory Christian International
PASTOR: Apostle Carl White

Kyahna Haine was diagnosed with Hodgkin's Disease Lymphoma at age 18. She went through multiple rounds of Chemotherapy for about two and one half years. At the age of 22, the cancer finally went into remission and Kyahna was able to start living her life again.

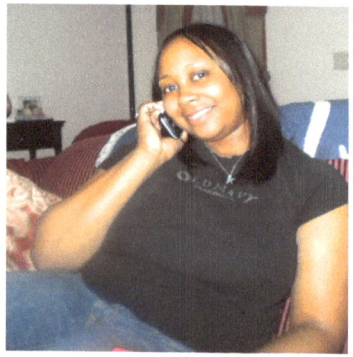

BEFORE

At this point, she was very thin and frail from the chemotherapy but she was alive and joyful. Kyahna wasted no time living again, re-enrolling in college and spending as much time with her family and friends as she could. She really wanted to enjoy life so she started eating every meal like it was her last.

Kyahna had a part time job at Olive Garden. She found herself snacking on breadsticks and other things from the menu on every break, even though she wasn't necessarily a fan of the restaurant's food.

Outside of work, Kyahna had a sedentary lifestyle. Her claim to fame is that she wouldn't walk to her mailbox if she didn't absolutely have to — and her mailbox is next to her front door!

It took only a few years of this behavior for Kyahna to find herself at 5'4" and more than 180 pounds! She never knew exactly how much she weighed because, she says, "Who weighs themselves when they are really fat?!"

She became disgusted with her appearance. She wouldn't shop for clothes because she had to be so picky about what she would wear so the clothes wouldn't show her fat rolls — and she had more rolls than a bread basket at Red Lobster.

It was around this time that her sister, Carlene, suggested they attend a workout class at their church. They had both heard on the radio about a Personal Trainer (that's me!) who was touring churches and making health and fitness presentations while at the same hosting different boot camps. He was going to be at Victory Christian International Ministries — their church — soon.

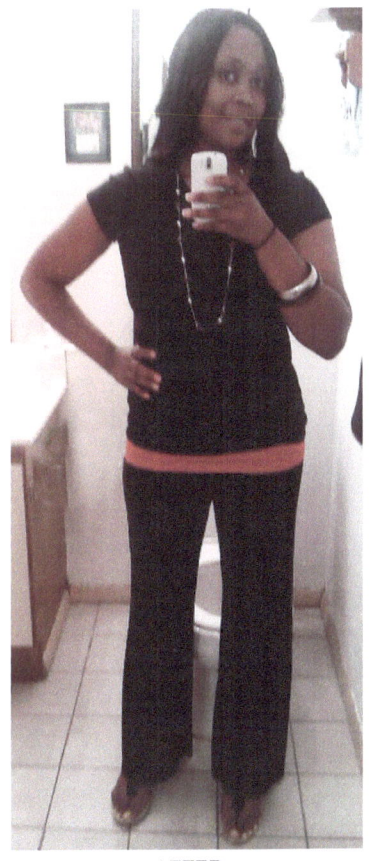

AFTER

While she was attending my classes, I would assist Kyahna by telling her what foods to eat and which ones to stay away from. I also encouraged her to start jogging because it would be something easy for her to fit into her schedule. Kyahna instantly bought new running shoes and got so into jogging that she started including most of her friends.

She became a pseudo personal trainer, encouraging all of her Facebook friends to start exercising and even took them to the gym with her. In three months, Kyahna was down two dress sizes and was more toned than she'd ever been.

Armed with the knowledge I'd given her, Kyahna hopes to continue her healthy lifestyle and eventually encourage everyone in her family to be Fit 4 Life!

KYAHNA'S DIET OPTIONS:

BREAKFAST:
- High fiber oatmeal, multi-grain Toast & apple
- Yogurt and raw granola & banana
- Grapefruit and multi-grin toast

LUNCH:
- Subway turkey sandwich (no Condiments) w/ veggies
- Apple Cajun chicken breast, broccoli, nectarine
- Chicken or steak fajitas w/ whole grain tortillas/wraps (no condiments)

DINNER:
- Baked fish with mixed veggies
- Baked chicken, spinach, baked sweet potato
- Chicken tenderloins with multi-colored peppers, onions and mushrooms, fresh green beans, whole grain rice
- Lean steak w/cabbage
- grilled chicken
- Turkey breast w/wild brown rice

Forbidden Fruit

"The devil don't mind killing you with a biscuit or cocaine"

— APOSTLE AARON ROYSTER NEW JOY DIVINE

"He who keeps the law is a discerning son, but a companion of gluttons disgraces his father."

— PROVERBS 28:7

The Bible is a holy book filled with prophecy and law. Throughout the scripture, you can find instructions for what to do and how to do it. How then is it possible for Christians to be so confused about what to eat and how to eat? It's not the book's fault! The Bible gives actual instructions for this, but most Christians aren't paying attention and continue to be confused.

If I told you that I made my very own car from scratch and that it runs on unleaded fuel and nothing else. Would you believe me? Of course, you would! That's a reasonable thing to say you've done. If I were the maker of the car, then I would know what it needed to run and function properly at its optimum level. Well

God created man from the dust of the earth, so he is the maker of man.

Satan's first lie

Then the LORD God formed a man from the dust of the ground and breathed into his nostrils the breath of life and the man became a living being.

— GENESIS 2:7

Genesis 2:7 states that God is the maker of the human body. God did not create the body and breathe life into it without giving us instructions for how to get the most out of it. With this creation came distinct instructions on what fuel it needs to perform at optimum levels. God makes it clear in Genesis what foods we are to eat and what foods to stay away from. He not only suggests foods for humans to eat, but actually makes it a law not to eat certain foods as we read further along in the scripture.

Every moving thing that liveth shall be food for you; As the green herb have I given you all.

— GENESIS 9:3

The key to the above verse is, "As the green herb". There are many green herbs, including poison ivy, hemlock and deadly nightshade, but God doesn't want us eating poisonous green herbs. This verse is saying to eat of the land that which is good for you and not that which is bad for you.

When you see laws in modern society they are always enacted to create order and preserve life. The speed limit is 55 mph, because if every car drove 75 mph there would be chaos on the road and a plethora of accidents. A licensed gun carrier is the only one who can carry a gun legally because not everyone can use a gun without killing themselves and other people. So, laws are put into place so society can be controlled and everyone has a chance to live a full, healthy life.

The reason that many Christians today do not adhere to what is stated clearly in the Bible regarding what to eat and not to eat is because of the influence of Satan, the devil, Lucifer, the son of the morning ... whatever you want to call him. The scripture John 8:44 refers to the devil as "the father of lies". This means that you cannot trust what he says regarding anything.

What is the first lie the devil ever told to man? He lied about what to eat! In the scripture, food was the measuring stick of truth where Adam and Eve faltered. They both ate of the tree of Good and Evil, even though God told them not to. They didn't just eat it because they wanted to, they were deceived and actually encouraged to eat. Their disobedience not only cost them eternal life, it caused God to change what the devil would eat as well.

> **"The Lord God said to the serpent,**
> **"Because you have done this, cursed are you above all livestock and above all beasts of the field; on your belly you shall go, and dust you shall eat all the days of your life."**
>
> — GENESIS 3:14

The word dust means remains or decay and has a slang origin that actually means *to kill*. God limited the devil to only foods that would kill him when he ate them. Kill in this context doesn't mean instantaneous death, instead it's a slow, prolonged death where one must endure a sustained misery.

This description sounds all too familiar to me. When I talk to clients who had been overweight for years and then dropped all of the excess weight, I ask them how they feel. They almost always describe their old body as a prison and talk about how uncomfortable they were all the time. The devil's objective is for men and women to be just like him.

When we use the term devil here, we are referring to the polar opposite of God Almighty. When you look at a reflection of the word Devil in the mirror, it reads Lived. The devil is death and God is life!

THINK ABOUT IT

The foods in the garden was there to give Adam and Eve eternal life. Foods rejected by the garden were the foods that Satan feasts on. Most of those rejected foods were scavenger animals that feed on the remains of other animals — *not* fruits and vegetables.

CLEAN vs UNCLEAN

> *Among the animals, whatever divides the hoof, having cloven hooves and chewing the cud—that you may eat. Nevertheless these you shall not eat among those that chew the cud or those that have cloven hooves: the camel, the rock hyrax, the hare, and the swine, though it divides the hoof, having cloven hooves, yet does not chew the cud, is unclean to you.*
>
> — LEVITICUS 11:3-8 (NKJV)

These you may eat of all that are in the water: whatever in the water has fins and scales, whether in the seas or in the rivers—that you may eat. But all in the seas or in the rivers that do not have fins and scales, all that move in the water or any living thing which is in the water, they are an abomination to you.

— LEVITICUS 11:9-10 (NKJV)

Can you eat anything that you want to eat, as a Christian, according to the Bible? Absolutely not! There are foods that God strictly forbade and other foods that he did not. I have a created a list below that outlines what foods are considered clean by God according to the Scripture and what foods are unclean and shouldn't be eaten.

CLEAN MEATS:

ANIMALS: cows, sheep, goats, deer.

BIRDS: chicken, turkeys, geese, ducks, doves.

SEAFOOD: salmon, trout, and those fish with fins and scales.

UNCLEAN MEATS:

ANIMALS: pigs, horses, camels, rats, cats, dogs, snakes, raccoons, squirrels, most insects.

BIRDS: eagles, sparrows, crows.

SEAFOOD: catfish, sharks, scampi, octopus, squid, shellfish, and whales.

Unclean meats affect the human body negatively in a number of ways, including diarrhea, profuse sweating, muscle soreness and pain, and even prostration. You should eliminate unclean meats from your diet immediately. Some doctors will tell you, "There is no need to remove certain foods from your diet."

THINK ABOUT IT

Most doctors *do not* have healthier or longer life expectancies than their patients.

OLD TESTAMENT vs. NEW TESTAMENT:

"Do not think that I came to destroy the Law or the prophets. I did not come to destroy but to fulfill. For assuredly, I say to you, till heaven and earth pass away, one jot or one title will by no means pass from the law till all is fulfilled."

— MATTHEW 5:17-18

If the Bible says not to eat certain foods, then how do Christians justify eating them? Have you ever noticed that a pastor may reference the Old Testament when it comes to tithing and offerings but when the subject of food comes up the statement, *"We are under the new covenant,"* gets thrown around. The word tithe isn't even mentioned in the New Testament of the Bible but church members are still encouraged to do it.

When a pastor discusses the new covenant, he is referring to the Law of Moses and is saying that under the New Covenant, Christians do not always have to operate under the Law of Moses because they are allowed to operate under grace, which came about after the coming of Jesus. Usually, though, that same grace is not allowed when it comes to homosexuality or divorce. My question to them pastors is this, *"Do we follow the Bible or don't we?"*

Jesus did not eat pork or any other food forbidden in the Old Testament. We know this because he was raised under Jewish custom and law, which forbids the eating of certain foods. The carcass of the pig was not even touched by Jews; it was considered that foul and disgusting.

> **"But, I have this against you:
> You tolerate that woman Jezebel, who calls herself a prophetess, and by her teaching deceives my servants to commit sexual immorality and to eat food sacrificed to idols"**
>
> — REVELATION 2:20

What foods was Jesus talking about, if anything could be made available to eat? He was talking about foods that were considered *the remains* of real food, aka the leftovers. Understand that when discussing forbidden foods in the Bible this isn't just an "opinion" of what to eat and what not to eat. Foods that the Bible has stated should not be eaten have been proven over the years to have an adverse effect on one's health.

Here is a short list of some of the effects of eating foods that are forbidden in scripture:

- obesity
- heart attacks
- emotional imbalance
- difficulty in controlling sex drive

- the creation of blockages to higher logic
- weakens long-term self-control
- OCD **(Obsessive–compulsive disorder)**
- acne

THINK ABOUT IT

Trikinosis or trichiniasis trikinisis is a parasitic disease caused by the roundworm Trichinella spiralis this parasite is transmitted by eating raw or inadequately cooked meat, especially pork. The larvae are released, reach maturity, and mate in the intestines, then larvae are produced. The parasites are then carried from the gastrointestinal tract by the bloodstream to various muscles where they become encysted. It is estimated that 10% to 20% of the adult population in the United States suffers from trichinosis at some time.)

TRICHINOSIS – FROM *ENCARTA ENCYCLOPEDIA*

Many people say, "Anything can happen to anyone and everyone." That same person doesn't understand the mindset that comes along with discipline. You can never become a disciple without discipline, they go hand and hand. Following a leader requires the ability to follow instructions. The closer one aligns himself with instructions the more he becomes like his leader.

The head of the body of Christ is supposed to be Jesus Christ. How can we claim to be Christians and not be like or at least attempt to be like Jesus? Everyone has heard the saying, "You are what you eat". If you define yourself as a follower of Christ, that following must include dietary choices.

Jesus answered, "It is written: 'Man does not live on bread alone, but on every word that comes from the mouth of God.'"

— MATHEW 4:4

The scripture does not say that man will not live without bread (food) but that he will not live on food alone. One of the most important aspects of life is eating. Eating not just spiritual food but physical food, too.

When one's diet is contrary to the diet of God then unnecessary problems can and will arise. To think that problems with one's physical, emotional, and spiritual health are unrelated to what one is physically feeding oneself is absurd.

When you were sick as a child, your parents didn't say, **"Well, okay, just eat this candy and feel better. I know you like candy."** Your parents knew to give you soup, orange juice, lemon slices in tea, etc. They didn't have to go to medical school to figure out that sickness is best fought by healthy eating.

God is a loving parent who is very concerned with what His believers eat. He makes this clear in the Bible. He understands that any sickness you have or will get can be removed or avoided by healthy eating.

"A people who continually provoke me to my very face, offering sacrifices in gardens and burning incense on altars of brick; who sit among the graves and spend their nights keeping secret vigil; who eat the flesh of pigs, and whose pots hold broth of impure meat; who say, 'Keep away; don't come near me, for I am too sacred for you!' Such people are smoke in my nostrils, a fire that keeps burning all day."

— ISAIAH 65 3-6

The Sins of the Father

"You shall not bow down to them or worship them; for I, the LORD your God, am a jealous God, punishing the children for the sin of the fathers to the third and fourth generation of those who hate me"

— EXODUS 20:5

According to the Center for Disease Control (CDC), during the years 1980–2008 obesity rates doubled for adults and tripled for children. These numbers mean that almost 1.5 million American children are overweight.

Christian children outdo their Christian parents by being *more* overweight than non-church attending children. A young person does not construct his or her diet, parents do. Therefore, Christian parents are guilty of destroying the next generation with their lack of focus on physical fitness and healthy eating as it related to the Gospel.

Parents are feeding their children as if they were adults. Kids today are becoming addicted to sugar, junk foods and fast foods, the same way a crack baby is addicted to cocaine. The first rule of parenting is modeling — displaying the behavior you would like your child exhibit so that they mimic it. Using this behavior, we can expect overweight/obese parents to produce overweight/obese children. Even parents who are not overweight or obese but still have unhealthy lifestyles will most likely produce a overweight/obese children.

Portion size at fast food restaurants contain too many calories for most adults, so just imagine the effect they have on a small child's short- and long-term health. Plus, fast food today has more sugar and fat than ever before add that to the increase in portion size and parents really need to pay attention to what their child is eating.

Studies suggest the hormones used to produce meats cause increases in hormones in our young girls and boys, making them more prone to being overweight at an earlier age.

I was in a church service the other day and started to quietly cry when I saw a little girl who was so overweight that she was out of breath playing with the other children. The little girl was only 5 years old and she was so much bigger than the other kids that she couldn't even play with them. Someone is guilty of something, because that little girl did not make herself that big.

> **It would be better for him to be thrown into the sea**
> **with a millstone tied around his neck**
> **than for him to cause one of these little ones to sin.**
>
> — LUKE 17:2

A study done at UNC and published in The Journal of the American Medical Association *found: Between 1977 and 1996, portion sizes increased for salty snacks, desserts, soft drinks, fruit drinks, French fries, hamburgers, cheeseburgers and Mexican food. ... the quantity of salty snacks increased by 93 calories, soft drinks by 49 calories, hamburgers by 97 calories, French fries by 68 calories and Mexican food by 133 calories.*

Those numbers are even higher today. It's going to take mature, faith-filled parents to understand that we are not talking about different body types and a kid being cute and chubby. We are talking about the difference between a child living a healthy, normal life and a child experiencing premature death. The power of life and death today is not just in the tongue but also the teeth, the throat the stomach etc. The effect of being overweight as an adult is extremely difficult and it is magnified for a child.

EFFECTS ON A CHILD

Low self-esteem is the biggest problem for an overweight child. It has been shown in countless studies that overweight kids are more susceptible to bullying. They feel different from other kids in a negative way. They have a harder time participating in school activities for fear that other kids will make fun of them.

Many overweight kids live a life of severe depression, and oftentimes their parents fail to notice. When I was in high school, I watched overweight girls who had straight As in every class choose to make poor grades in the class and not to dress for gym class for fear of being made fun of. It is unfair for any child to grow up feeling shame about his or her physical appearance.

Daytime sleepiness is another serious issue that affects overweight children. When a child is overweight, countless studies show that it is more difficult for the child to stay awake during the day.

The majority of learning for young people takes place during the day. If a child does not have the energy to stay awake in class, how could they have the energy to focus? This problem affects everything from grades to physical development. A well-rested child even develops better physically than a kid who is tired all day.

Overweight children are bigger than their normal weight counterparts, but they are more susceptible to injuries because of their size.

The number of children who remain obese in adulthood is quite high. It is a fact that without significant intervention, 90% of individuals who are overweight by the age of 18 will remain so throughout their adult lives.

This person can pay a staggering price for being overweight. The actual cost of obesity over the course of a lifetime is likely to be $549,907.35 (according to Wellspring Camp for childhood obesity), with health insurance. That is over half a million dollars! Talk about starting your kids off with debt.

Poor health may follow an overweight child or the rest of his or her life.
"An overweight or obese child who develops Type 2 Diabetes by age 15 may be looking at kidney failure, heart attack or severe neurological damage by their 30th birthday"

— DR. DAVID LUDWIG, WHO LEADS A WEIGHT-LOSS PROGRAM, BOSTON CHILDREN'S HOSPITAL.

Obese children are at risk for a number of conditions, including:

- High cholesterol
- High blood pressure
- Early heart disease
- Diabetes
- Bone problems
- Skin conditions such as heat rash, fungal infections, and acne

You've probably heard the joke about the overweight mother who takes her overweight child to the doctor. The doctor tells the mother, "Your child is carrying too much weight to be so young. She needs to lose weight."

The mother replies, "It's okay. It runs in our family."

The doctor comes back with, "The problem is *no one* runs in your family!"

Poor health generational curse

A Christian parent has the spiritual authority to break the generational curse of obesity in his child's life. It will take honesty on the part of the parent and a firm resolve, but with faith put into practice, it can work. It is no secret that the effect of overeating and being lethargic in children is eroding our society from a health care standpoint. The worse part about this epidemic amongst Christian youth is that they cannot lead from the backseat.

As individuals who have given their lives to the Lord, our young people should not only be the moral examples but the physical examples of what the kingdom produces. That is not the case currently.

> **Fathers shall not be put to death for their children,
> nor children put to death for their fathers;
> each is to die for his own sin.**
>
> — DEUTERONOMY 24:16

Most parents have become enablers, feeding their kids the same things they eat, and allowing their children to sit in front of video games or the television all day. Then they wonder why the child is tired and physically and mentally exhausted. It's because of all the greasy food that sits in his/her stomach! Just remember the old adage, "You are what you eat."

> **Direct your children onto the right path,
> and when they are older, they will not leave it**
>
> PROVERBS 22:6

THINGS TO ELIMINATE FROM A CHILD'S DIET

SUGAR — Parents should do their best to eliminate sugar from a child's diet. Parents should moderate their child's consumption of candy, cookies, cake and sodas on a daily basis. These items are okay for special occasions but shouldn't be a regular part of a child's diet. (The weekend shouldn't be considered a special occasion.) The good thing about eliminating these foods from a child's diet is that the less they eat of these foods, the less they crave them. Ever heard of putting sugar in a gas tank to lock up the engine? Well, the same holds true for children and their attention spans. Too much sugar makes it more difficult for a child to concentrate.

TRANS FATS AND SATURATED FATS — Avoid high concentrations of trans fats and saturated fats. These fats inhibit healthy brain and nerve functioning, which can lead to the development of ADD (Attention Deficit Disorder) symptoms. Saturated fats directly raise total and LDL (bad) cholesterol levels. Trans fats are used to extend the shelf life of processed foods, typically cookies, cakes, fries and donuts. Any item that contains "hydrogenated oil" or "partially hydrogenated oil" likely contains trans fats. This unhealthy fat raises our bad cholesterol levels while lowering the good ones. This contributes to heart disease. Parents should opt for healthier alternatives such as olive oil, canola oil and flaxseed oil. Keep in mind that all fats have 9 calories per gram, compared to 4 calories per gram for carbohydrates and proteins. Remember, just because you're avoiding trans fats by eating low-fat brownies, doesn't mean they're calorie free - they can pack a big calorie punch that can also lead to obesity.

FRUCTOSE AND GLUCOSE — One key reason for avoiding foods and beverages containing high fructose corn syrup has to do with the type of sugar contained in the sweetener. High fructose corn syrup contains an average of 55 percent fructose and 45 percent glucose, whereas table sugar has a 50-50 ratio. This difference may seem slight, but to a child's body it is significant. Fructose does not stimulate the secretion of insulin, which helps regulate ones blood sugar. Fructose and Glucose are directly related to obesity and Type 2 Diabetes. The key to avoiding these types of sugars is to keep young people away from fast food restaurants all together. Almost everything on these menus is high in high fructose corn syrup — from the drinks to the buns. This means home cooked meals have to be made on a regular basis.

Would a Man Rob God?

"By 2030, obesity could account for more than $860 billion in health care expenditures"

— JOURNAL OF THE AMERICAN MEDICAL ASSOCIATION

"... a sinner's wealth is stored up for the righteous."

— PROVERBS 13:22

The Church has to be at the forefront of the fight against obesity and obesity-related diseases. For the Church to be most effective, it has to start with the pastor and make its way down. Over $40 billion a year is spent on weight loss products.

It is time for the church to capitalize on life, not death. Yes a fried chicken dinner could mean a few extra dollars towards the building fund, but the long-term effects are ravaging the capital that can be generated by the body of Christ.

Imagine what the church would look like if "Divine health" was focused on more than "Divine healing". Being overweight or obese is the most expensive thing a person can have in his or her life. The solution for physical wellbeing can be found in the gospel. If the church can repent and turn away from its ungodly practices then there is a small fortune awaiting the body of Christ.

Some may say that you shouldn't sell health, but those same individuals would never protest McDonald's or Burger King selling death in the form of high calorie food! These billion dollar companies make their living by making the believing community fat, which leads to them becoming out of shape, tired, and sick.

Have you seen the movie *Supersize Me?* There is a guy who goes on an all McDonald's diet and almost dies from it within 30 days. Instead, you should go on an all fruit and vegetable fast for 30 days and tell me how you feel afterward.

Below is a short list of how churches can change their formats to start appealing to the longevity that was promised to the Christian community at large in the Gospel.

- **ENCOURAGEMENT.** The best way to curb obesity is through encouragement. Pastors and clergy should bring up the issue on a regular basis instead of pretending it doesn't exist. People who are overweight should be talked to in a loving and compassionate way and encouraged to be healthier. There should be counseling sessions in the church the same way Alcoholics Anonymous has meeting and receives funding. The church should be able to market its weight loss services as not only a way to save lives but also a way to save money.

- **INFORMATIVE SPEAKERS.** Bring in guest speakers from the health/fitness field. Having a fiery preacher come in on one Sunday as a guest is great for the morale of the church. Having a personal trainer, doctor or nutritionist come in and speak would be better for the long-term health of the group. Bringing in an accredited individual who knows what he or she is talking about would be of interest to everyone in the church and would go a long way towards educating the congregation.

- **TAKE IT OUTSIDE.** Initiate a walking plan for all members of the church or take the church out of the four walls. Go out into the community and pass out literature about the church. It's a great way to get exercise for the church members and also increase church enrollment. You might even bump into a few Jehovah's witnesses and Muslims while you're out there, because members of every religion are out there walking around — except Christians.

- **HEALTHY EATING.** Promoting healthy eating in the church. Stop trying to make a fast buck by bringing vending machines into the church or opening candy shops. Try bringing in fresh fruit and selling that instead. Maybe even open a healthy smoothie station and assign someone in the church the job of blending fresh fruit to be made available after church.

- **INVEST IN FITNESS.** Invest in a walk or bike path around the church or build a gym inside the church. When building a new church facility, plan for a nice area where members can walk and/or workout to increase their physical activity level. Having an area for members to workout would keep people at the church longer during the week. This also would bring non-church members to the church. People near the church will eventually want to stop by to see what's going on. This could lead to an increase in enrollment.

THINK ABOUT IT

"By 2030, obesity could account for more than $860 billion in health care expenditures"

— JOURNAL OF THE AMERICAN MEDICAL ASSOCIATION

Price/Cost/Worth

How many times has the church had to take time to pray for a sister or brother because they're in the hospital because of diabetes, hypertension, heart attack, stroke, or any other obesity or poor health related disease? What's often overlooked is how often that same person is one of the biggest contributors to the Church. Most times, they aren't.

When they're in the hospital, they aren't paying tithes or making offerings. When they get out of the hospital, they have a lot of bills to focus on, so they reduce their tithes and offerings. By noticing this, I'm not being selfish, I'm being real.

"Will a man rob God? Yet, you rob me.
"But you ask, 'How do we rob you?' "In tithes and offerings.'

— MALACHI 3:8

Below are some eye-openers about the costs of being overweight and out of shape.

KNEE INJURY: One of the most common injuries an overweight person will experience is knee. This injury is so common that I've never trained an overweight person who didn't have a knee injury. If one has insurance and injures his knee and requires an MRI, surgery, and physical therapy, it could cost about $2000 out of pocket $2000 in a year.

SLEEP APNEA: Overweight and out of shape people have a hard time sleeping. With insurance to cover visiting a sleep lab, sleep prescription pills, and a c-pap machine, one could end up paying $1000 in a year.

FOOD: It shouldn't be a secret that overweight people eat more than thin people. There are big people who would not like to admit it, but they do eat more. With eating more, they have to spend more. Being just 30 pounds overweight means spending an extra $10,000 more a year on food.

LIFE INSURANCE COSTS: Normal weight — $3,254 Obese — $3,924 Severely obese — $5,695 (*Business Week's* average numbers for life insurance per year)

FROM THE JOURNAL OF THE AMERICAN MEDICAL ASSOCIATION (JAMA) AND CENTER FOR DISEASE CONTROL AND PREVENTION (CDC)

Other eye-opening information to consider if you're overweight:

- You're less likely to be married and more likely to be divorced
- You're less likely to hold managerial jobs
- You'll spend more out of pocket on medical costs ($10,000 on average)
- You'll spend more on diet items (with lower likelihood of success)
- You'll spend more money on clothes
- You'll suffer from self-esteem and body image issues

HOW MUCH IS YOUR HEALTH WORTH?

BLOOD PRESSURE: The more you weigh, the higher your blood pressure. Besides possibly causing a stroke or heart attack, high blood pressure can lead to blindness and kidney failure. **How much are your eyes or your kidneys worth to you?**

CANCER: The liklihood for every type of cancer is increased by 50% when a person is overweight. There is a five times greater chance of getting gallbladder cancer for men and women who carry extra weight. **What is a cancer free body or a body that can survive cancer worth to you?**

TYPE 2 DIABETES: 85% of Type 2 Diabetes cases are overweight people. Here is a short list of the effects this disease: blindness, amputation, kidney and nerve disease, etc. I wouldn't give up one of my legs for $30 million. **What is being able to walk and keep your limbs worth to you?**

Fast Food is not cheaper

Fast-food companies spent $4.2 billion on marketing in 2009. This group wants people to eat on the go and to eat fast-food. They've even created a lie that eating healthy is expensive and eating fast food and junk food is cheaper.

I was teaching an exercise class in a church the other day. After class, a lady told me she wanted to eat healthy but she and her family just couldn't afford it.

A recent *New York Time*s article titled "Is Junk Food Really Cheaper" completely dispelled this myth. It showed that you can serve a family of four to six people a roasted chicken with vegetables, a simple salad and milk for about $14, In contrast, a meal for the same people at McDonald's — for example, two Big Macs, a cheeseburger, six chicken McNuggets, two medium and two small fries, and two medium and two small sodas — costs about $28.

As well as costing more, you have to also understand that fast food is not as filling as a home-cooked meal, so you need more of it to actually get full. This is basically junk food, and junk food is empty calories. That's why you can eat an entire bag of chips and still be hungry, but eating two apples makes you extremely full.

The world would have you thinking that you're saving money by running to a fast food restaurant or grabbing something quick from the vending machine. I reality, you're wasting money, eating empty calories and ruining your health.

PERSONAL STORY #3

Talyia

CHURCH: Trinity United Church of Christ
PASTOR: Otis Moss

Talyia embarked upon her endeavor to be "Fit 4 Life" while getting ready for her wedding. She thought it might be "cute" to lose a couple of pounds before her wedding. She never realized that by hiring "The Personal Trainer", i.e. me, she was beginning a radical change to her body, appearance, and overall health.

At that time, she wore a plus size 24 and was probably tipping the scales at 300 pounds, though she can't say for sure. She was initially so ashamed of her obesity, she wouldn't weigh-in. She'd been working out with me for about three weeks before she had the courage to weigh herself.

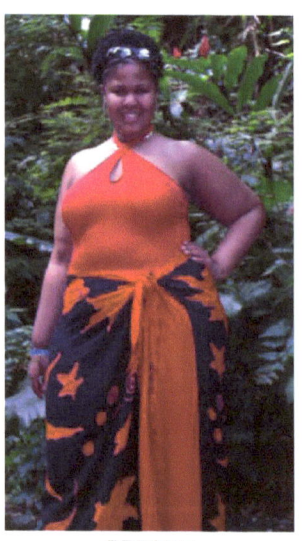
BEFORE

When she finally stepped onto the scale, it read 286 pounds. At 5'10", she wore the extra weight better than the average 5'7" woman, but she was still dangerously overweight.

One of the first changes she made in her diet was to eliminate red meat. Several years prior to this, as a Lenten sacrifice, she had given up red meat, so she knew she could do it. Next, she cut out fried foods completely.

As the pounds continued to fall off, she was motivated to make even more changes. She switched from caramel in her coffee to sugar-free vanilla and stopped using sugar to sweeten beverages.

Around the time she lost her first 50 pounds, I asked her to keep a Food Diary, which she loved doing. I told her to record everything she put in her mouth in a notebook, and to avoid snacking. Talyia found that because she didn't want to write down anything "bad," she exercised extreme discipline.

Today she is slim and trim and garners plenty or attention in the gym due to her fit physique.

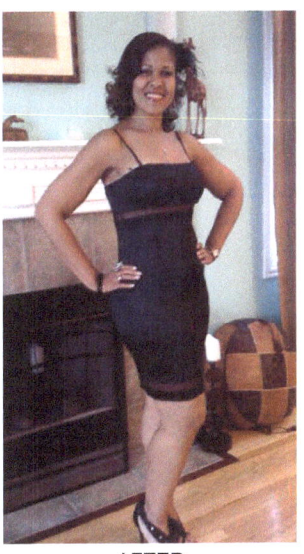

AFTER

TALYIA'S EXERCISE ROUTINE:

3 days weight training

3 days cardio

6 days total (every week)

FAVORITE CARDIO: Elliptical

TALYIA'S DIET (TYPICAL DAY):

BREAKFAST:
Coffee w/sugar-free caramel and soy milk, one banana

LUNCH:
One apple, strawberries, mandarin oranges and a Spinach Salad or peanut butter and jelly sandwich

DINNER:
Tilapia and couscous or salmon with a sweet potato and broccoli

SNACK:
Pecans, diet coke

FAVORITE FOOD:
Guacamole

Building Solomon's Temple

"When I get put in the ground everything on me will be exhausted"

— APOSTLE R. D. HENTON

Physical training is good, but training for godliness is much better, promising benefits in this life and in the life to come."

— 1ST TIMOTHY 4:8 "

Physical exercise should be part of every Christian's daily schedule if God says it's good. I need you to really understand how God sees the word "*good*". In Genesis 1:31, it says that on the sixth day of creation, when God had created everything looked at all He'd created and saw it was good. Good to God is great to man.

The physical vessel that harnesses a believer's soul should be held in higher regard than his or her home or car. Spending two hours waxing your car but not dedicating anytime during the week to exercise is a grievous sin. Having a body that is aesthetically pleasing is not vanity based; it is showing respect for what is given and a high regard for the giver.

God gives us legs to use as much as we can, arms to use as much as we can, a stomach that balances out our body, and a list of other body parts that are to be exhausted upon our departure from the earth. Have you ever heard the phrase, "Whatever you don't use, you will lose"?

From a physical standpoint, this is saying is particularly true. The technical term for not using your body is *Disuse Atrophy*. This happens when a muscle loses its strength, tone and elasticity because it is under used. This usually takes place with people who don't exercise and live a sedentary life. As this happens to them, they become physically weak, more prone to sickness and disease, and increasingly lethargic.

This condition is easily reversed by starting an exercise program. The most obvious problem with the Body of Christ is defining what exercise is and then actually doing it.

> *"But those who trust in the LORD will find new strength.*
> *They will soar high on wings like eagles.*
> *They will run and not grow weary.*
> *They will walk and not faint."*
>
> — ISAIAH 40:31

TYPES OF EXERCISE

CARDIO — The word Cardio means heart. **More than 910,000 Americans die of heart disease every year.** According to some studies, performing cardio (jogging, walking, jumping rope, elliptical, stairmaster, etc...) *30 minutes a day, 5 days a week* can reduce your risk of fatal heart disease by more than 75%. Cardio helps you control your weight and can reduce your chances of developing other conditions that may put a strain on your heart, such as **high blood pressure, high cholesterol and diabetes**. It also reduces stress, which is another major factor in heart disease. The best way to stay consistent with your cardio routine is to find a partner to perform your cardio with. Exercise like praise is not something that you should do alone.

> **"For where two or three come together in my name, there am I with them"**
>
> — MATHEW 18:20

The benefits of Cardio exercise go well beyond just the physical. The mental state of a believer is affected a great deal by performing cardio on a daily basis.

> **"For where your treasure is, there your heart will be also."**
>
> — LUKE 12:34

Cardio activity stimulates brain chemicals that will leave you feeling happier and more relaxed. I've noticed that after a really good run, I'm too exhausted to really argue with anyone, about anything. You may also feel better about your appearance and yourself when you exercise regularly, which can boost your confidence and improve your self-esteem.

THINK ABOUT IT

My sister Halimah always says, "If you look good, you feel good and if you feel good then you look good"

"Cardiovascular health is more important than any other single factor in preserving and improving learning and memory."

— THOMAS CROOK, PH.D.,
CLINICAL PSYCHOLOGIST AND MEMORY RESEARCHER.

With physical education being cut out of school programs, jobs requiring less and less physical activity, performing cardio has become more critical today than at any other time in history. There will always be an excuse for not starting a cardio routine but the key is to fight through the excuses and do it.

Be sure you are ready for the workout. Purchase a comfortable pair of workout shoes. Knee injuries are common if you're overweight or you don't have the right shoes. This injury will set any believer back and keep him or her from accomplishing the goal.

The ideal time to perform cardio is first thing in the morning before you eat. The reason for this is because your body will burn more fat when your stomach doesn't have protein or carbs to burn.

RUNNING vs. WALKING — Which is better for you, running or walking? I get this question a lot. Both are exercises are natural motions, which means you don't have to be taught how to do them. The one that's right for your workout will depend on you.

There isn't a better or worse here, just different. Walkers will tell you "running is bad for you" and runners will tell you "walking isn't really a workout." Both are technically right and both are also wrong.

Answer the questions below to determine which exercise is best for you:

1. ARE YOU OVERWEIGHT? There is a weight chart on my website, www.cf4life.com/weight. Check it to see where you are. If you're overweight by 20 pounds or more, running is a bad idea. *Why?* Because of the pressure it puts on your knees and joints. If you're not overweight, start off with light jogging if you've never run before, it will really benefit your cardiovascular endurance.

2. HOW OLD ARE YOU? If you're under 35 with no serious injuries, walking is unacceptable as a form of cardio. You're just too young to do the same workout as my grandmother — I'm sorry. So, all those people who are hitting the trail with big mamma walking, you need to pick it up — and I'm not talking about a sandwich.

3. HOW MUCH TIME DO YOU HAVE? If you only have 30 minutes on your lunch break, then you obviously can't run 3 miles because you have to get back to work. If you have 30 minutes *after* work, then you need to run. If you run for 20 minutes or walk for 50 minutes, you end up burning about the same amount of calories. But if you walk for 20 minutes or run for 20 minutes, running will create the biggest calorie deficit.

STRETCHING — Knee pain, lower back pain, difficulty with exercise, etc. can all be attributed to a lack of flexibility. A believer should be stretching every single day, even if it's just touching toe-touches in the morning before going to the bathroom. Each stretch should be held for 15-20 seconds.

For a list of stretches, visit **www.CF4LIFE.com**.

Stretching is one of the most important things you can do for your body. I've had clients live with joint pain and other painful areas for years, only to have that pain disappear within two weeks with consistent stretching.

> *"And the Egyptians will know that I am the LORD when I stretch out my hand against Egypt and bring the Israelites out of it."*
>
> — EXODUS 7:5

Benefits of Stretching:

- **INCREASED FLEXIBILITY AND JOINT RANGE OF MOTION**

    Flexible muscles can improve your daily performance. Tasks such as picking up a baby, bending to tie your shoes or hurrying to catch a bus become easier and less tiring. From age 20-70, the average person will lose 70% of their range of motion. That loss can be offset with daily stretching.

- **IMPROVED CIRCULATION**

    Stretching increases blood flow to your muscles. Blood flowing to your muscles brings nourishment and gets rid of waste byproducts in the muscle tissue. Improved circulation can help shorten your recovery time if you've had any muscle injuries. My flexible clients (Steve Zuckerman, Edward Calahan, Mary Mohr, etc.) have been back in the gym within days after an injury. My clients who are less flexible, however, can be out for weeks or even months from the same injury.

- **BETTER POSTURE**

    Frequent stretching can help keep your muscles from getting tight, allowing you to maintain proper posture. Good posture can minimize discomfort and keep aches and pains at bay. When a believer stands upright, it attracts non-believers to them. Standing straight with shoulders back is a display of royalty, as in the case of Saul the King of the Israelites.

- **STRESS RELIEF**

    Stretching relaxes tight, tense muscles that often accompany stress.

- **ENHANCED COORDINATION**

    If you feel a lack of balance, it's most likely due to a lack of flexibility in your muscles. Maintaining the full range-of-motion through your joints keeps you in better balance. Coordination and balance will help to keep you mobile and less prone to injury from falls, especially as you get older.

RESISTANCE TRAINING — There is only one way to become spiritually stronger and that is through life resistance. There is also only one way to become physically stronger and that is through resistance training — lifting weights, resistance bands, push-ups, sit-ups, squats, lunges, etc.

> *"He is the God who girds me with strength and prepares my ways."*
>
> — PSALMS 18:33

Resistance training builds the body up in a positive way and helps to fight against disease and depression, and gives you strength to function in everyday life.

Having strong muscles stands out in every culture around the world and is a public display of discipline. There is a difference between strong muscles and big muscles. The idea that to be strong one has to become physically massive is ridiculous.

Women tend to shy away from resistance training because they feel their muscles will become too big and they will start to look manly. That is one of the biggest myths in resistance training. Women can lift consistently heavier weights every single year and maintain a slender, feminine physique. If you don't want to look like a man, shave the mustache but keep lifting the weights!

Men can use resistance training to fight against belly fat and build a strong body. Young people can use resistance training to improve in sports. The elderly can use resistance training to increase body density. There is no single group that doesn't benefit from a regular resistance training routine.

How much resistance training is enough?

Resistance training should be performed anywhere from 2-4 times per week. One body part shouldn't be highlighted during a resistance training workout. There is something called ***opposing muscle group***. This is the muscle that is on the opposite side of another muscle. When someone only works just their stomach or chest muscles, it is usually to the detriment to the opposing muscle group. This is also how injuries happen.

Correct form is extremely important when doing a resistance training program. I suggest that everyone hire or work with a fitness professional initially to learn more about resistance training and proper technique. I once knew a chiropractor that looked for new business in a gym because he could tell from bad exercise technique who would soon be in need of his services.

There are some people who will shy away from resistance training and attempt to lose weight through fad diets and/or cardio only. This is a huge mistake! The benefits of resistance training go far beyond weight loss. Everyone stands to benefit from lifting weights, doing push-ups, or any other exercise that puts pressure on the muscles and joints.

> *"Have I not commanded you?*
> *Be strong and courageous! Do not tremble or be dismayed,*
> *for the LORD your God is with you wherever you go."*
>
> — JOSHUA 1:9

THINK ABOUT IT

According to the American Heart Association, moderate weight lifting offers benefits for those with heart disease or a family history of heart disease.

Here is a list of some of the many things that resistance training do:

- **INCREASE BONE MINERAL DENSITY** — Human bones are not fragile, but do weaken with age. From about 30 years of age on, the average person loses strength in his or her bones. This is why it's a lot easier for an elderly person to break a bone than it is for a 25 year old. To increase the strength of your bones, some stress must be placed on the bone. Resistance training puts enough stress on the bone to stimulate the bone density, therefore making it stronger.

- **INCREASE STRENGTH** — A muscle is able to grow when pressure is put on it. I've had clients come to a training session and before the session begins they'll tell me how weak their arms are. I always ask them same question, "How often do you exercise your arms?" Their response is always the same, "I don't." Each time you attempt to lift or pull something it puts pressure on your muscle. Your muscle responds to this pressure the same way your spirit does, by getting stronger. There is no limit to the growth of the human muscle. This means a person can get as strong as he or she wants. With greater strength comes greater sacrifice. To do 50 push-ups at one time may only take about 10 minutes a day, depending on what fitness level you're at when you start. As your number of push-ups increases, the time you require for training will increase, too.

- **INCREASE THE RANGE OF ACTIVITIES** — When your body is strong enough to lift considerable weight, you will also be capable of doing more strenuous activities. If you want to run a marathon, it's possible, but your body has to be strong enough to withstand the stress on your joints. Being able to withstand stress on your physical body will translate to other activities in your life.

- **REDUCE BODY FAT** — Using and increasing your muscle mass (even a little bit) will increase the energy required by your body, even at rest. This also increases the energy needed by your body at during activities. The more muscle, the more energy it takes to supply your body so it functions properly. This translates to more fat calories and fat being burned each minute. Thus, with the decrease in body fat, you can expect the tone of your body to improve and you will become leaner. A woman who weighs 150 pounds and has 19% fat will look much smaller (and be much healthier) than a woman weighing 150 pounds with 35% fat. They weigh the same amount, yet their composition is different. Because muscle is denser than fat, the person with less fat and more muscle will look smaller.

- **IMPROVE THE STATE OF THE ELDERLY** — For the elderly, maintaining a resistance training program will help improve health and decrease the risks brought on by the age. If you've noticed that your grandparents are getting shorter over the years, it's because of the lack of strength in their lower back and core area. Elderly can be more independent if they keep their muscles strong. Imagine an 95 year old who needs no help walking or doing things in his or her daily life. Who says 90 is too old to do whatever you want? We live in a society where 30 year old people are caring for 60 year olds because they can't do it themselves. That puts a tremendous stress on our culture.

- **IMPROVED HEART CONDITION** — Regular resistance training can result in a lower heart rate and lower blood pressure, especially after exercise. Thus, the risk of heart diseases is reduced. The heart is a muscle just like the biceps. As stress is put on the heart, it becomes stronger. This actually increases a person's chances of survival when undergoing surgery. It most instances, it's not the disease that kills, it's the treatment. Their heart isn't strong enough to survive the surgery or treatment for the actual disease and that is the reason they die.

Resistance training, when properly done, will change your physical, emotional, and spiritual life. I always stress this to Christians, "How do you expect to get on your knees and ask God for anything if you can't get down on your knees?" God did not create us to be victims, to walk around half crippled and unable to carry our own groceries to the car at 40 years of age. He intended for us to be victorious.

Believers mentioned in the Bible were strong, not just in faith but physically as well. Caleb was a believer who came to Moses with a good report on entering the Promise Land. He was an old man who was said to have the strength of a young man.

> *"Finally, be strong in the Lord and in his mighty power."*
>
> — EPHESIANS 6:10

BONUS CHAPTERS

Top 10 Gym Mistakes

"All Scripture is breathed out by God and profitable for teaching, for reproof, for correction, and for training in righteousness"

— 2ND TIMOTHY 3:16

1. **NOT STRETCHING** — If you want to get leaner, faster and have a better-looking body, stretching assists with all of those things. A tight muscle is not just begging for an injury, it will always be underdeveloped. In a test of the 1976 Olympic team for flexibility, gymnasts were ranked number one and power lifters were ranked number two. **Stretching also makes you stronger!**

2. **NOT SETTING REALISTIC GOALS** — Unrealistic and vaguely stated goals are among the leading causes of exercise dropout. The key is to establish a training goal that is specific and appropriate for your fitness and skill levels—something a bit challenging but not overly difficult. "To look good" is not a goal. "To drop one pound per week for the next 10 weeks through exercising six days a week" *is* a goal!

3. **BAD FORM** — I hate it when I walk into a gym and see guys who think they're the strongest people on earth because they grab heavy dumbbells and do an exercise with terrible form! They're not really even exercising and they'll eventually hurt themselves. Extend your arms or legs fully and retract them fully, none of that half stuff.

4. **THE ALL-OR-NOTHING APPROACH** — Not having a full hour to exercise is no reason to skip your workout. Research shows that even 10 minutes of exercise can provide important health benefits.

5. **NOT BALANCING YOUR TRAINING** — Regardless of your goals, you should have a balance of both cardio and strength training. Even if you're looking to lose weight, you should perform strength training (muscle incinerates calories). If you're looking to build muscle, you should also exercise your heart with cardio.

6. **EXERCISING TOO HARD** — If you've skipped several workouts, don't try to make up for lost time in one session — you're only setting yourself up for soreness and a possible injury. There are no make-ups: just start where you are.

7. **WRONG WORKOUT PARTNER** — having a workout partner who is too fit or too fat compared to you. When you go to the gym and your workout partner doesn't motivate you or worse, discourages you, the results won't be good. The same will happen if your workout goals are different. It will not work! Find someone who is close to where you are and trying to go where you're headed.

8. **SAUNA SUIT PEOPLE** — Everyone has seen the person in the gym who is working out using some weird gimmick to try to speed the process. They're wearing a sauna suit or garbage bag, are wrapped

in plastic wrap or they're wearing one of those ridiculous stomach sweat belts. We've all laughed at that person. Look, the only thing any of those items do is make a person lose water weight. There are no shortcuts to success! Work hard and eat healthy every day and you'll get the results you want.

9. **DOING THE SAME THING** — The best exercise for you is a different exercise today than you did yesterday. Variety is not only the spice of life, but the key to real results. You can find new workouts on the internet, in magazines, or by working with your personal trainer. Just please, do something different.

10. **BEING A POLITICIAN** — The gym is not the place to launch your political campaign or work on your stand-up comedy routine. If you go to the gym and try to talk to everyone about everything, then you will never get any real results. A ten-minute conversation may not seem like much, but when your gym time is limited, losing those 10 minutes will throw off your workout completely — trust me, I know first-hand.

Water — the liquid of life

But those who drink the water I give will never be thirsty again. It becomes a fresh, bubbling spring within them, giving them eternal life.

— JOHN 4:14

The word water is mentioned in the Bible over 700 times. If God felt a need to use one word that many times, shows how really be important it is. The Bible starts off in *Genesis 1:2: Now the earth was formless and empty, darkness was over the surface of the deep, and the Spirit of God was hovering over the waters.*

God chose to position his very own spirit over water in the beginning of creation. The question is why? Reading this chapter you will help you to understand how the most important part of our health and fitness program has been given to us in the scripture but has been constantly overlooked by the believer.

A human being can live for weeks without any food but can only live a few days without water. It has been shown that if you lose just 2.5% of your body weight from water loss, you will lose 25% of your efficiency. The human body is anywhere from 55% to 78% water depending on body size. A rule of thumb is that two-thirds of your body consists of water, and it is the main component of human body.

Here is where the water is:
- Muscle — 75% water
- Brain — 90% of water
- Bone — 22% of water
- Blood — 83% water

The functions of water in human body are vital and include:
- Transport nutrients and oxygen into cells
- Moisturizes the air in lungs
- Helps with metabolism
- Protect the vital organ
- Helps the organs to absorb nutrients better
- Regulates body temperature
- Detoxifies
- Protect and moisturizes the joints

Water and Christ are synonymous in the scripture, so to be a true believer one has to be physically hydrated. Water isn't a question of like or don't like, it's more a question of Life and Death.

Instead of water, Christians have been attempting to hydrate themselves with high fructose corn syrup. Beverages containing high fructose corn syrup have high levels of reactive carbonyls, which are linked with cell and tissue damage that leads to diabetes.

You can find high fructose corn syrup in soft drinks, sports drinks, lemonades, iced tea, and almost every sweet drink you can think of. In 1970, Americans consumed less than a pound of this syrup per year. By 2005, the average was 42 pounds, according to the *Seattle Times*.

Have you noticed that if you drink a glass of water and then drink soda pop right after it, the soda pop tastes funny? The reason for this is because those drinks are exact polar opposites of what we're supposed to consume to hydrate ourselves. They serve two completely different functions in the body and don't work together at all.

> **"No servant can serve two masters..."**
> — LUKE 16:13

If you're not drinking water throughout the day or you don't like water at all, then your body is suffering because of it. Eight out of 10 believers are dehydrated. You may be dehydrated as you're reading this and not even know it.

> **Whoever believes in me,
> as the Scripture has said,
> streams of living water
> will flow from within him."**
> — JOHN 7:38

What is the best water to drink

There are so many different water options on today's market that it's easy to understand how one can become confused. Some waters are safer than others and some taste better than others.

> *"Let us draw near with a true heart in full assurance of faith, having our hearts sprinkled from an evil conscience, and our bodies washed with pure water."*
>
> — HEBREWS 10:22

Here is a list of what's really behind certain H_2Os:

DISTILLED WATER — This is nothing more than boiled water that has been allowed to condense. Distilling is a method of purification that is used to remove solid particles from water. This is the cheap version of mineral water.

MINERAL SPRING WATER — Spring water is a type of bottled water that comes from under the ground and flows naturally to the earth's surface. According to FDA regulations, to qualify as spring water the water can't be collected anywhere except at the site of the spring.

TAP WATER — Water that comes from your faucet — tap water — is not to be trusted. Many of the pipes that this water flows through are what make it unsafe. Also, chlorine is used to disinfect the water, and we all know where else chlorine can be found — swimming pools. You don't want to drink a pool.

BOTTLED WATER — If it doesn't say spring water, don't drink it. Many of the bottled water companys just repackage tap water and throw a fancy label on it. Also, waters like Dasani add salt to make the consumer thirstier so they'll drink more water.

How much water should you drink?

All water flows from life and as believers if we expect to have an abundance of life. If we want this, we must focus our minds on consuming an abundance of water. The question always comes into play, **"How much water should I be drinking?"** As a rule of thumb 8-10 glasses is generally accepted, but I disagree with that number because everyone's physical activity and body weight is different.

For example, Person A delivers mail in Georgia and weighs 250 pounds and Person B weighs 150 pounds and is a computer programmer who works in an air-conditioned office. ***Do you think they need the same amount of water per day?*** Absolutely not!

The most obvious reason for the difference is that Person A loses a lot more water during the day through sweating from being outside and from physical activity.

> **When the poor and needy seek water, and there is none, and their tongues faileth for thirst, I the LORD will hear them, I the God of Israel will not forsake them. I will open rivers in high places, and fountains in the midst of the valleys: I will make the wilderness a pool of water, and the dry land springs of water.**
>
> — ISAIAH 41:17-18

When figuring how much water you're consuming, you must also factor in that there is plenty of water in fruits and vegetables which add to the amount of water that you consumer per day. I tell my clients to keep water around all the time —in your purse, office desk, refrigerator, everywhere you are. Attempt to drink it steadily throughout the day and you will be okay.

Fruits and vegetables with high water content

96% — Cucumbers and Iceberg lettuce. Add both to a salad and have before you eat lunch or dinner.

95% — Tomatoes, zucchini, radishes and celery. Also, vegetables that should be added to a salad. They can be found in soups as well.

92% — Eggplant, cabbage, cauliflower, sweet peppers, spinach, strawberries and watermelon. Eggplant Parmesan, strawberry daiquiris, sautéed spinach and roasted cauliflower can be prepared at home any day of the week.

91% — Grapefruit and broccoli. Eat grapefruit raw in the morning. Add broccoli to salads, casseroles, or eat steamed or sautéed.

> *"For I will pour water on the thirsty land,*
> *and streams on the dry ground;*
> *I will pour out my Spirit on your offspring,*
> *and my blessing on your descendants."*
>
> — ISAIAH 44: 3

Water dictates how one's body moves and functions. It also affects how one thinks and one's energy level. Until drinking enough water becomes a part of a person's daily routine, health will always be an elusive thing. Not having enough water can cause short-term memory problems, increase trouble with basic math, and cause problems focusing on smaller print like that found on a computer screen.

Drinking enough water on a daily basis can decrease cancer risk including colon cancer by 45% and bladder cancer by 50%, and it can potentially reduce the risk of breast cancer. The more water one drinks, the better one feels physically and spiritually.

The body of Christ needs to make water available to the believers in the same way that fried chicken and collard greens have been made available. Water is a drink that should be allowed within the sanctuary of every church. There must be an aggressive movement amongst believers so that anyone who desires to drink more water can have it made accessible in Jesus' name.

When you are experiencing low energy, fatigue, excess weight, poor digestion and aches and pains it may be attributed to the pH Balance in your body being out of order. How does the pH Balance get out of order? *This like processed sugar, meats, dairy, coffee, alcohol, etc. create an acid ash in the body. This acid can be likened to the oxidation that takes place when fruit when left out or when metal rusts. It eats away at our bodies and ages us faster than normal.*

THINK ABOUT IT

Nine out of 10 Americans are dehydrated right now and even those who are hydrated aren't getting the most out of the water they drink.

Just to give a further idea of the importance of water in our diets, to survive, the body can stand to lose the following:
- 50% of your glucose
- 50% of your fat

- 50% of your protein; but
- but only 20% of your water!

HOW WATER HELPS YOU LOSE WEIGHT

- Water maintains proper kidney function, which increases the efficiency of the kidney's fat burning ability

- Water acts as an appetite suppressant, when the average person feels hungry they are really just dehydrated

- Water intake reduces water retention, I know this may sound crazy but it actually does

- Water helps improve the efficiency of a workout by helping your body perform at optimum level

- Water increase your energy throughout the day, because most people have never been hydrated they don't realize the difference it makes in energy level

Sleep is the Cousin of Death

*"It is vain for you to rise up early,
to sit up late, to eat the bread of sorrows:
for so he giveth his beloved sleep"*

— PSALMS 127:2

It has become common practice for believers to stay up all night and watch TV or even participate in vain conversation. *Sleep is one of the most important things a person can do for his or her health.*

Everything good that can happen to the body will happen as a result of getting full night's rest. Sleep promotes physical health, longevity, and emotional wellbeing. Without adequate sleep, judgment, mood, and ability to learn and retain information are diminished.

A Christian should end every day in prayer followed by a full night's rest (at least most nights out of the week). I understand that sometimes things come up and you may need to work through the night, that's fine, just don't make it a habit.

Here are some interesting facts about sleep deprivation:

- The National Highway Traffic Safety Administration (NHTSA) estimates conservatively that each year drowsy driving is responsible for at least 100,000 automobile crashes, 71,000 injuries, and 1,550 fatalities.

- Sleep deprivation induces significant reductions in performance and alertness. Reducing your nighttime sleep by as little as one and a half hours for just one night could result in a reduction of daytime alertness by as much as 32%.

- It has been estimated that lost productivity at work due to sleepiness at work may cost the US economy as much as $100 billion annually.

It is recommended that a person get anywhere from eight to nine hours of sleep a night, but most of us don't even get seven. Rats deprived of sleep die within two to three weeks, a time frame similar to death due to starvation.

Whether you exercise on a regular basis not, sleep is of extreme importance to you. During sleep your body produces the most growth hormone, therefore, the more sleep you get the faster your muscles will heal and recover from your workout.

Below is a list of conditions that have direct links to lack of sleep:

- Heart attack
- High Blood Pressure

- Heart failure
- Stroke
- Obesity
- Psychiatric problems, including depression and other mood disorders
- Attention Deficit Disorder (ADD)
- Mental impairment
- Fetal and childhood growth retardation
- Injury from accidents

That extra hour or two you spend watching late night TV could be your last extra hour or two! If sleep is the cousin of death, then not getting enough sleep is the drunk uncle who lives in the basement. Look at these numbers and you will understand why getting a good night's rest is the best thing you can do for your health, fitness, and even your pocketbook!

Under the Influence

"Don't be drunk with wine, because that will ruin your life. Instead, be filled with the Holy Spirit,"

— EPHESIANS 5:18

Drinking alcohol is not in and of itself a sin according to the Bible, but drinking alcohol in excess *is* a grievous sin. So, what is excess? *(Excess is defined as: the state or act of going beyond normal, sufficient or permitted limits).*

Anyone who drinks or has drunk alcohol knows and understands the concept of *alcohol tolerance*. Tolerance is how many drinks a person can have before alcohol affects his or her decision-making ability or becomes flat-out drunk.

There is a debate about this amongst believers because a person who has been drinking isn't necessarily qualified to judge, how much control he or she does or doesn't have. In many Scriptures, alcohol is attached to a list of immoral things.

"Because we belong to the day, we must live decent lives for all to see. Don't participate in the darkness of wild parties and drunkenness, or in sexual promiscuity and immoral living, or in quarreling and jealousy."

— ROMANS 13:13

Drinking any amount of alcohol can easily lead to drinking it in excess. Because of the possibility of becoming offensive, exercising poor judgment and/or causing the stumbling of others, the best choice for Christians is mostly likely to abstain from drinking alcohol.

Additional Reasons Not to Drink

1. **ALCOHOL SUPPLIES ALMOST TWICE AS MANY CALORIES AS PROTEIN & CARBOHYDRATES**

   One gram of alcohol contains seven calories. This is much more than the four calories that are found in one gram of carbohydrate or protein. It is a bit lower than the 9 calories contained in a gram of fat, but considering how many grams of alcohol can be found in a bottle of beer or a glass of wine or a shot of Vodka, you'll see that by drinking alcohol, you're adding a ton of calories to your diet.

2. **ALCOHOL LOOSENS THE INHIBITIONS**

   This effect is one reason why people tend to seek out alcohol in social situations, but also can cause people who drink to keep drinking more than is wise and to eat a lot of extra food that they shouldn't have had in the first place. This adds even more calories to your diet creating an indirect calorie surplus, which can cause weight gain quite easily.

3. **ALCOHOL CAN DAMAGE THE STOMACH, KIDNEYS, AND LIVER**

   Alcohol essentially poisons the organs. The liver may eventually become inflamed resulting in alcoholic hepatitis, which can result in scarring of the liver (isn't that right?), liver failure and death. Alcohol can cause the stomach to become inflamed as well (gastritis), which can prevent food from being absorbed and increase the risk of cancer.

4. **ALCOHOL LOWERS TESTOSTERONE**

   Testosterone, which has a powerful fat-burning effect, is reduced whenever alcohol is consumed, thus halting its full potential. Also, testosterone is an anabolic hormone, which means that it contributes to gains in lean muscle mass. Lowered testosterone means fewer muscle gains, and less muscle means a lowered metabolic rate.

5. **ALCOHOL INCREASES APPETITE**

   Researchers from Denmark 's Royal Veterinary and Agricultural University have shown that if a group is given a meal and allowed to eat as much as they wanted, alcohol, rather than a soft drink, would increase the amount of food consumed.

www.ingramcontent.com/pod-product-compliance
Lightning Source LLC
Chambersburg PA
CBHW041219070526
44584CB00001B/14